boost
your
energy
naturally

For Denis, naturally

THIS IS A CARLTON BOOK

Text copyright © 2002 Beth MacEoin
Design copyright © 2002 Carlton Books Limited

This edition published by
Carlton Books Limited 2003
20 Mortimer Street
London W1T 3JW

A CIP catalogue record for this book
is available from the British Library

ISBN 1 84222 791 2

Printed and bound in Dubai

The author and publisher have made every effort to
ensure that all information is correct and up to date
at the time of publication. Neither the author nor the
publisher can accept responsibility for any accident,
injury or damage that results from using the ideas,
information or advice offered in this book.

The application and quality of beauty products,
treatments, herbal preparations and essential oils
is beyond the control of the above parties, who
cannot be held responsible for any problems
resulting from their use. Always follow the
manufacturer's instructions and, if in doubt, seek
further advice. Do not use herbal preparations
or essential oils without prior consultation with a
qualified practitioner or medical doctor if you are
pregnant, taking any form of medication, or if you
suffer from oversensitive skin.

Editorial Manager: Judith More
Art Director: Penny Stock
Senior Art Editor: Barbara Zuñiga
Executive Editor: Zia Mattocks
Design: Zoë Dissell
Editors: Siobhán O'Connor and Lisa Dyer
Production Manager: Janette Burgin

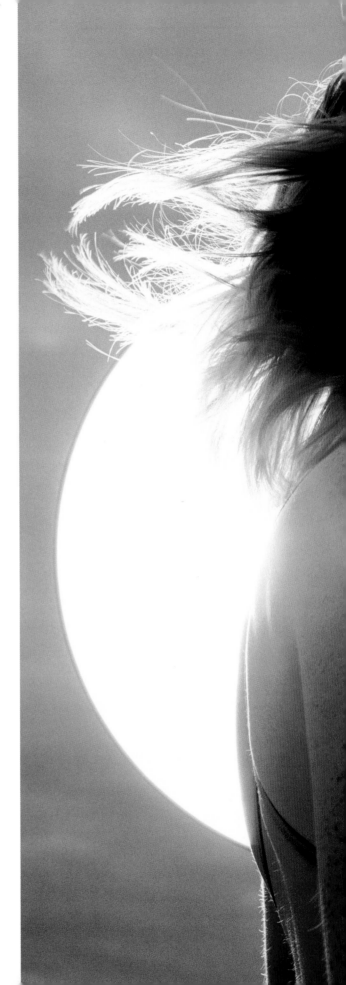

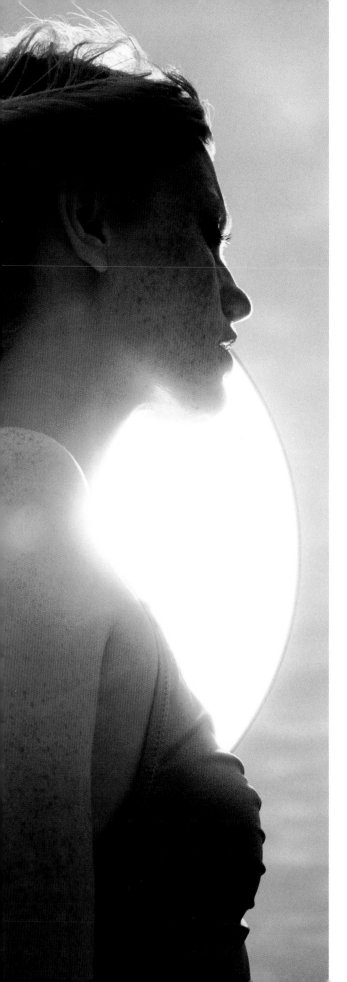

boost your energy naturally

THE COMPLETE GUIDE TO REVITALIZING YOUR BODY AND MIND

Beth MacEoin

CARLTON
BOOKS

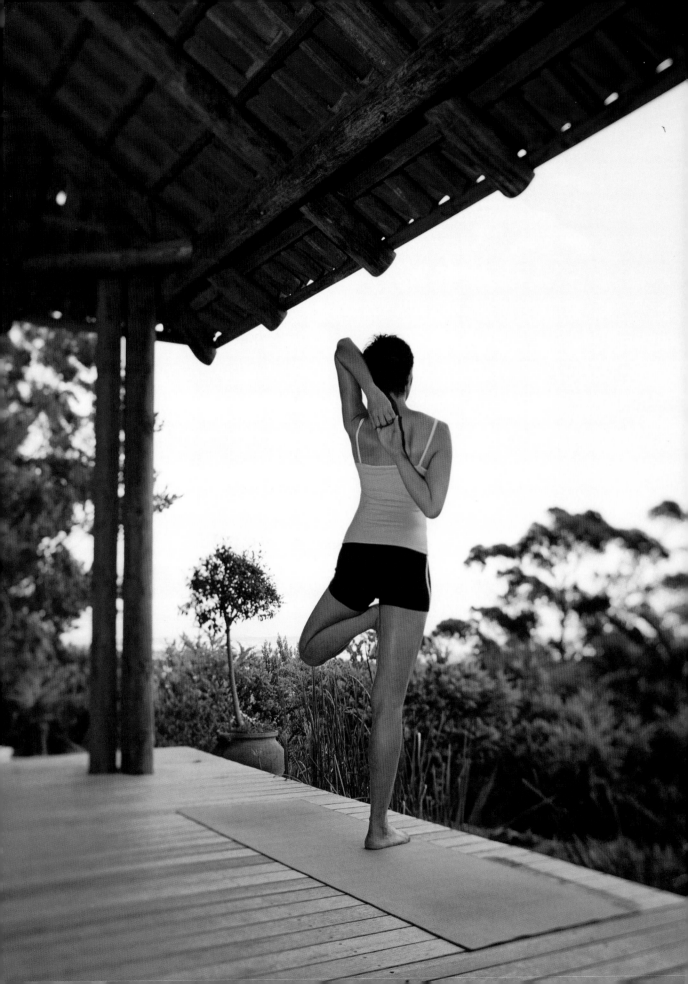

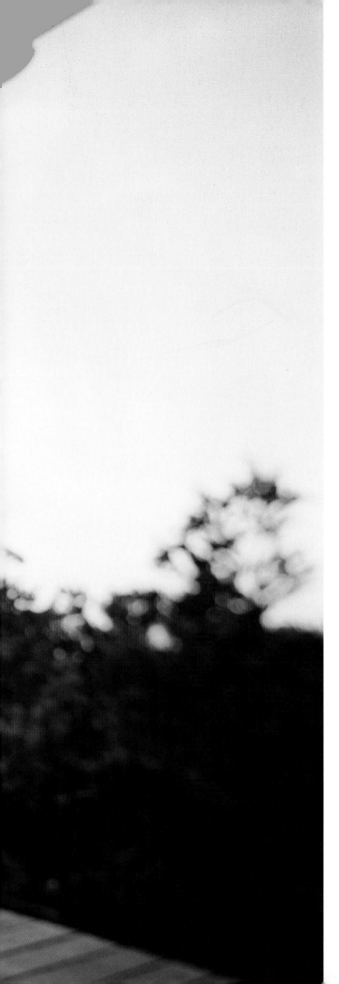

Contents

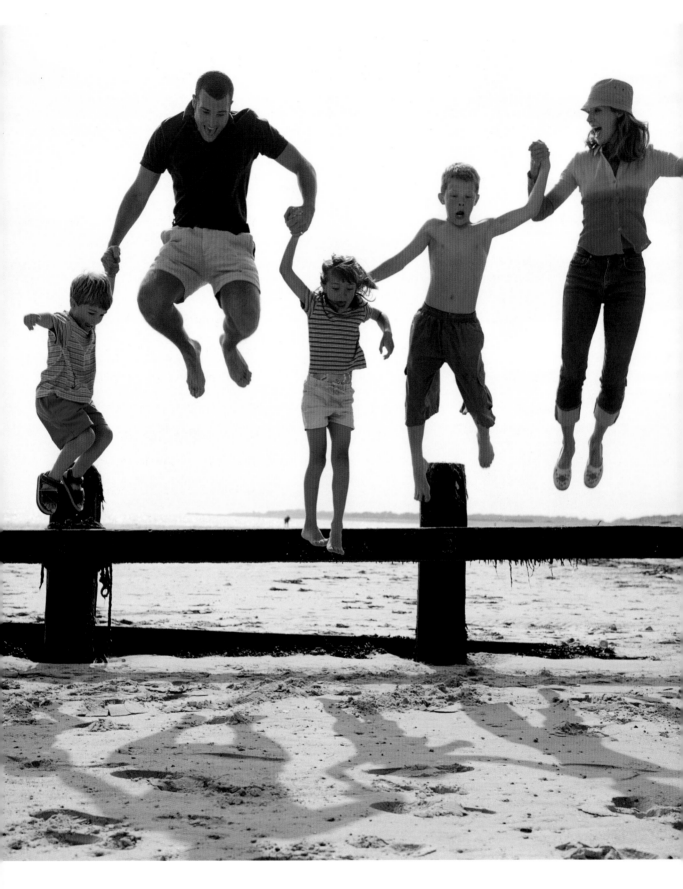

Introduction

Do you feel as though you are always 'running on empty'? Does pleasure pass you by because you feel constantly under par? Does your concentration wander when you try to focus on mental tasks? If you've answered 'yes' to any of these questions this book has been written with you in mind.

Healthy, smooth-flowing, balanced energy levels supply the spark of life. Who among us has not noticed that, when we're filled with a sense of emotional, mental and physical vitality, life flows so much more positively? Any problems that pop up – and, of course, it's in the nature of day-to-day life that they will – can be faced with confidence and resourcefulness when we are brimful of healthy energy. Yet the opposite is also unfortunately true. We are unlikely to be able to think creatively and laterally when we feel completely drained and exhausted.

These observations have significance for our personal relationships, as healthy levels of vital energy are important in helping us to make the most of the relationships that matter most in our lives. High levels of vitality enable us to enjoy the many pleasures that come from socializing with friends, playing with children, working and thinking creatively and making love. They also help us to maintain a healthy sense of humour in sticky patches.

Yet how many of us unconsciously settle for energy levels that can be best described as lacklustre? We know how stressful and demanding modern-day life has undeniably become, and, as a consequence, many of us may have given into the common assumption that life is simply an exhausting business.

This book is intended to help you to deal effectively with the obstacles that life presents from time to time, challenges that can leave us feeling less than dynamic. It also highlights the fact that you shouldn't be afraid to aim high to enjoy optimum levels of vital energy.

LEFT **HIGH LEVELS OF POSITIVE ENERGY SHOULDN'T JUST BE LIMITED TO HOLIDAY TIME. BY TAKING APPROPRIATE, ENERGY-BOOSTING MEASURES, YOU CAN MAKE THEM A REGULAR AND SUSTAINED FEATURE OF YOUR DAILY LIFE.**

Boost Your Energy Naturally aims to provide you with a workable, practical scheme that you can adapt to bring your basic sense of vitality back on track as quickly, effectively and easily as possible. Specific problem areas are identified in chapter one, while the chapters that follow provide a long-term plan designed to give the essential information you need to ensure that you don't 'crash and burn' again.

Most important of all, rest assured that this project isn't going to be a deadly solemn, punishing or Spartan business that fills you with dread at the mere thought of attempting it. *Boost Your Energy Naturally* has been consciously assembled with a view to making the changes suggested in it as accessible, rewarding and pleasurable as possible. It is my hope that you will find that, as more balanced energy levels return, you begin to discover a renewed sense of *joie de vivre*. I wish you fun and the best of health on your journey to enhanced vitality.

Don't forget that healthy energy levels are balanced energy levels. In other words, you should have plenty of vitality to meet the demands and challenges of everyday life, without moving on into a state of hyper-energy overdrive. If the latter occurs, although you may well feel in the short term that you are being superproductive, the odds are that you will pay a high price for this extreme behaviour in the health stakes later.

Operating in overdrive is definitely not good for your wellbeing in the long term. Living your life in fifth gear can make it very difficult for you to switch off and relax, with all sorts of health problems – most commonly tension headaches, migraines, digestive upsets and a poor sleep pattern – lurking just around the corner.

Instead, you should aim for a steady baseline of balanced emotional, mental and physical vitality that gives you the freedom to work, play and relax as you choose. In the long run, your body will thank you for it. Balanced levels of mental, emotional and physical energy are essential if we are to genuinely experience positive health and vitality. Apart from putting a bounce in our step and balancing erratic moods swings, healthy and stable levels of energy are an essential aid in supporting the basic bodily processes of repair, maintenance and cellular renewal. When energy levels are flowing smoothly we fight off minor illnesses more effectively as well as feeling as though we have an increased zest for life.

RIGHT **YOU CAN USE SIMPLE HYDROTHERAPY TECHNIQUES TO PERK YOU UP OR TO CALM YOU DOWN, DEPENDING ON YOUR INDIVIDUAL NEEDS AT ANY GIVEN TIME.**

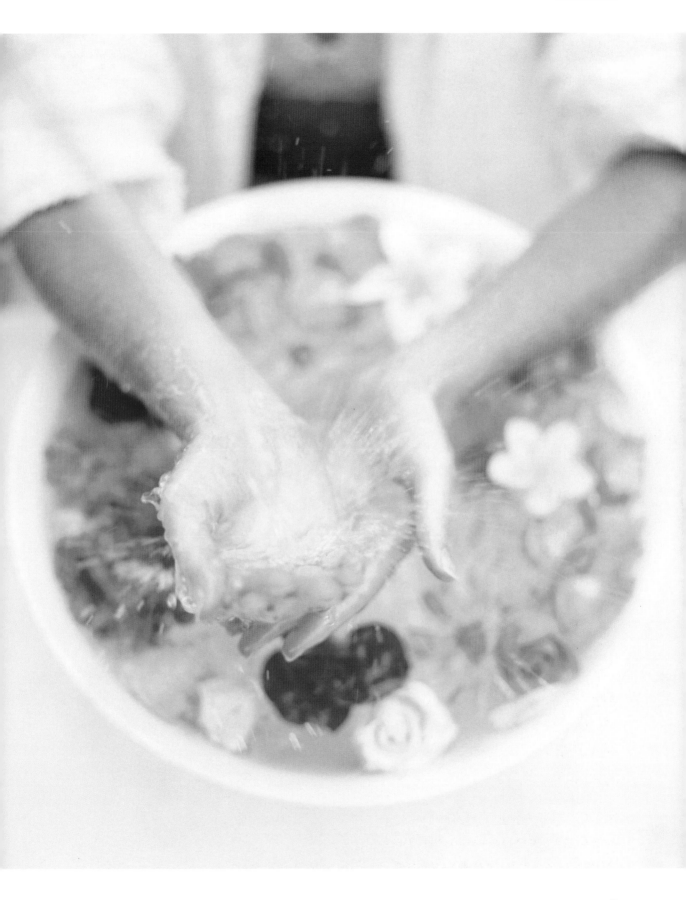

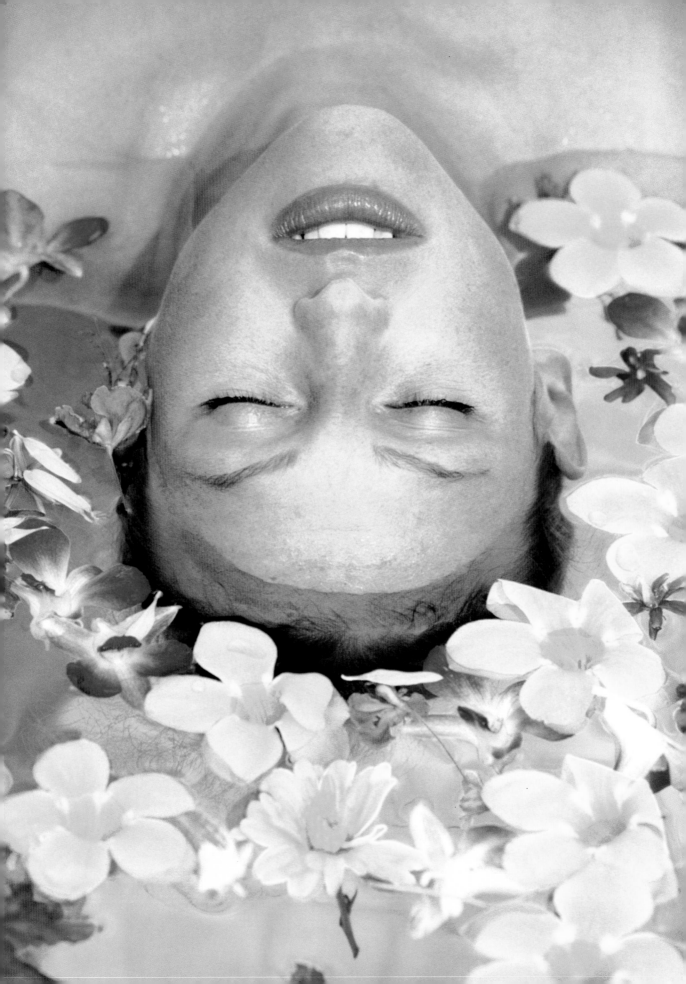

1 Energy medicine

These days it is difficult to open the pages of a glossy magazine without finding at least one feature on alternative and complementary medicine. Therapies such as homeopathy, acupuncture and herbalism, once considered fringe practices or just for cranks, have moved firmly on to centre stage, where they are increasingly accepted as popular and effective systems of healing. Many of us may have friends or colleagues who think nothing of having reflexology, aromatherapy or chiropractic treatment to help with tension headaches or back pain. It is also not uncommon now for enlightened GPs to suggest to their patients that they consult a homeopath or traditional Chinese therapist in order to treat their persistent eczema or psoriasis.

Perhaps the most telling indicators of alternative medicine's broad-based popularity are the shelves of the major pharmacy and supermarket chains. Here substantial and ever-increasing space is dedicated to medicines, nutritional supplements and 'natural' cosmetics stocked only by small specialist health food stores just a couple of decades ago. Once large-scale retail chains and department stores begin to devote significant amounts of space to these products, we can be certain that public interest and support for alternative medicines and therapies have grown to levels that should be considered significant.

Even the hardest-headed of us will soon find it difficult to ignore the fact that we have a wide range of non-conventional therapies at our disposal that can treat a multitude of debilitating and chronic conditions. What we may not yet have realized, though, is that alternative and complementary therapies possess an extra dimension that goes way beyond the effective treatment of a variety of common conditions that includes irritable bowel syndrome, migraine, anxiety, depression, arthritis, premenstrual syndrome and acne. This crucial extra dimension is related to a concept that lies at the heart of so many alternative and complementary therapies: the importance of stimulating vital energy.

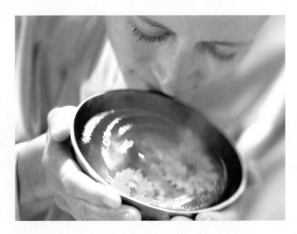

LEFT **HOLISTIC THERAPIES CAN HELP YOU TO DEAL WITH LIFE'S CHALLENGES GENTLY BUT EFFECTIVELY.**
RIGHT **MANY COMPLEMENTARY THERAPIES SUCH AS MASSAGE AND AROMATHERAPY ARE A PLEASURE IN THEMSELVES.**

VITAL ENERGY:
THE SPARK OF LIFE

Speak to any alternative therapist and you are likely to find that, once they begin to talk about the way in which their therapy works, they will invariably discuss the stimulation of healing energy. What is noticeable is that each therapist will use different words to describe the same basic thing. For example, a homeopath will talk about the vital force, while an acupuncturist will refer to *chi*. An ayurvedic practitioner will discuss the balancing of *doshas*, while a yoga teacher will be concerned with the stimulation of *prana*, or the breath of life. While the terminology employed differs in each case, each practitioner is talking about exactly the same thing: energy.

As a result, when these therapies are effective, they do much more than merely treat the symptoms of illness. Instead, they are thought to stimulate a profound experience of healing that goes way beyond the absence of symptoms. Most significant of all is that when they work to their maximum effect they have the potential effectively to balance our mental, emotional and physical levels of energy. And once this vital balance is established, a state of wellbeing emerges that you may have regarded as something lost forever in the dim and distant past.

It is precisely this capacity to stimulate healing energy that has given rise to much scepticism about many alternative therapies. After all, we cannot see with the naked eye the acupuncture points and meridians (the channels of energy believed to run along the surface of the body by practitioners of traditional Chinese medicine), any more than we can detect any molecules of the originating substance in a homeopathic remedy. However, even the sceptics are being forced to re-evaluate their views as tentative, plausible explanations are emerging that seem to offer vital clues as to what may be happening on a rational basis. The links that have been established between the secretion of endorphins (feel-good chemicals produced by the body) and the use of

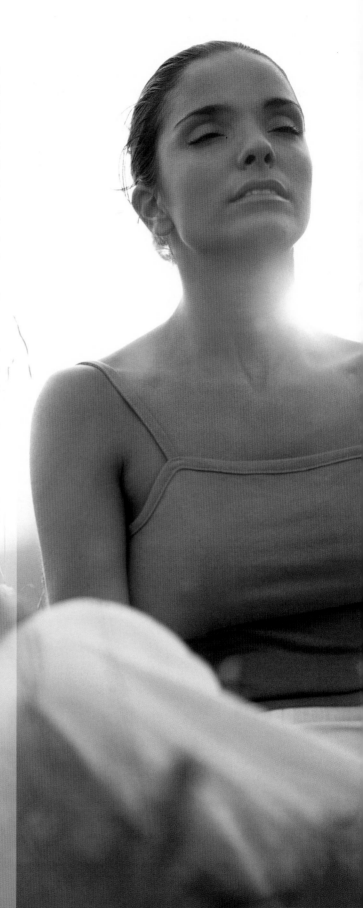

acupuncture have led some members of the medical establishment to consider the possibilities and validity of using acupuncture for pain relief.

There is still a long way to go before we have any hard-and-fast explanation for the way in which homeopathic remedies have such a dramatic curative effect when accurately prescribed, yet some interesting theories are being explored even in this controversial area. These include the 'memory of water' experiments, which suggest that water molecules may take the imprint of whatever substance has been used as a starting point in making a homeopathic remedy, so that the solution may still have the capacity to stimulate a positive healing energy response well after any of the molecules of the original substance have departed from the solution.

Don't worry: it's not the object of this chapter to become bogged down in abstract theory about the intricate workings of alternative and complementary medicine. This book's primary purpose is to provide a practical guide to the tools we can use to kick-start our energy batteries and keep them topped up. On the other hand, it is important to know that the therapies that form the foundations of the approach to healing described in the following pages do have some basis in scientific fact. It's just that the traditional parameters need to be expanded a little in order to make room for exciting, fresh possibilities in the growing area of energy medicine.

Now that we've briefly considered the developing field of non-conventional approaches to healing, it's time to take a closer look at the all-round benefits of stimulating a positive energy spiral.

LEFT **PRACTISING MEDITATION REGULARLY HELPS THE MIND TO SWITCH OFF AND IMPROVES CONCENTRATION.**
RIGHT **YOGA IS AN IMMENSELY POPULAR ENERGY-BALANCING, BODY-CONDITIONING SYSTEM OF MOVEMENT.**

ACHIEVING A POSITIVE ENERGY SPIRAL: THE REALITY

Once you've descended into a negative energy spiral, it can feel almost impossible to break free (for a general picture of this slippery slope, see the section on pages 15–16). Yet moving into a positive energy experience is very often only a step away: the trick is knowing where and how to break the negative behavioural cycle in which you may have become caught. Most of us nurse the best of intentions when it comes to exercising regularly, eating well and getting our sleep pattern into line. If you can't discover the positive impetus necessary to make a start, however, the chances are that you will keep putting off the action that you need to take. As a result, you'll probably feel guilty about not taking active steps to improve your situation, compounding the problems associated with the negative energy spiral into which you're slowly but surely descending.

One of the most effective ways of turning all those good intentions into reality is to find and embark on a suitable course of alternative or complementary treatment. This is because the energy-based systems of healing outlined on pages 21–31 aim to give your body's self-healing potential a boost. As a direct consequence, basic energy levels should rise proportionally. If treatment is successful,

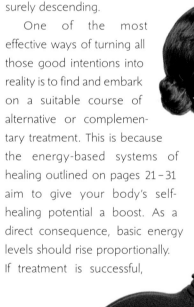

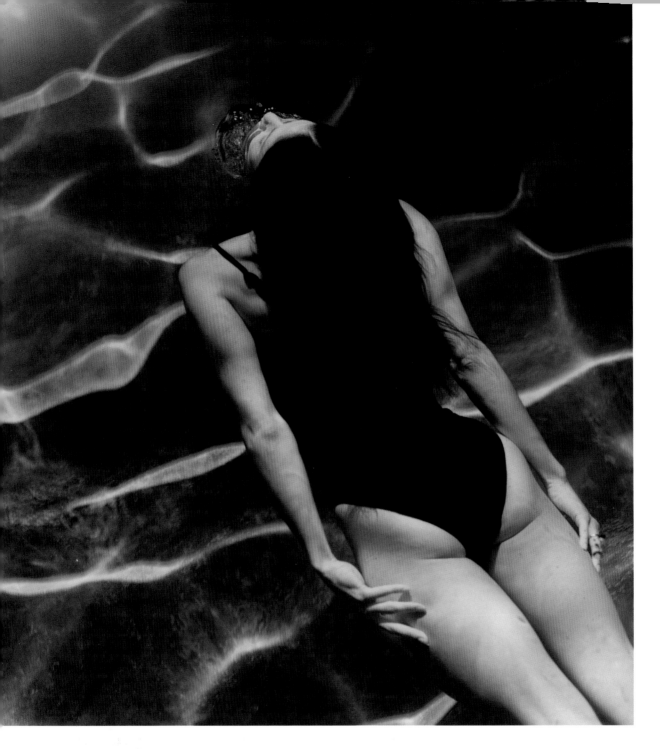

ABOVE **SWIMMING USES YOUR LARGE MUSCLE GROUPS AND CONDITIONS THE LUNGS, PROVIDING ALL-ROUND BENEFIT.**

the ensuing rise in your mental, emotional and physical vitality will be exactly what you need to give you a firm nudge in the right direction.

If you make the most of this energy boost, you are likely to find that you start to eat more healthily, eliminating quite happily the junk food that you have been wanting to jettison from your diet for months. Finally, getting to grips with this issue offers two advantages: taking positive steps towards enhanced health will give you a psychological boost, and you are also likely to discover that your improved eating patterns further improve your energy levels.

As this positive energy spiral climbs yet higher, you may feel ready to organize yourself to improve your physical fitness. The chances are that eating healthier foods, you will see the benefit in the loss of a few unwanted pounds. This encouraging sign can then inspire you to take up a form of enjoyable physical movement that will help you to develop a stronger, more flexible body shape. Regular exercise also has its own special effect on the body's chemistry, one that goes way beyond the purely psychological boost that comes from feeling more confident about your body strength and shape. It has been demonstrated time and again that rhythmic aerobic exercise stimulates the body to secrete endorphins. These naturally occurring chemicals have a profound effect on our brain chemistry, making us feel positive, calm and energized.

Once you've come this far, you are in a prime position to tackle some of the broader areas of your life with which you have been dissatisfied, but which may have seemed to demand too much of an effort to tackle when you felt drained of energy. Sorting out a muddled financial situation, leaving an unrewarding or unsatisfactory job, re-training for something you have longed to do for ages, getting to grips with a dependence on addictive patterns of drinking, eating or taking prescription drugs such as sleeping pills or tranquillizers, contributing more positive energy to a flagging relationship in order to revive it, recognizing that a relationship is going nowhere and finding the resolve to end it: all these scenarios need energy. Yet postponing them stops you moving on. Once you have the energy to tackle them positively, you are likely to feel an intense sense of liberation and a further boost of energy.

In short, then, as you reach the peak of your experience of a positive energy cycle, you are likely to feel more alive than you have for years. Don't be misled: this isn't some mystic state of nirvana where you reach a peak of enlightenment and will, thereafter, sail through life on a magic cloud for ever. Life will always throw all sorts of surprises at you, but once you have firmly laid down the foundations of a practical, energy-boosting plan, you should find that you can deal with these crises more effectively and bounce back again in double-quick time. Conversely, if you're heading for a negative energy cycle when crisis hits, coping with it may seem impossible.

EXPERIENCING A NEGATIVE ENERGY SPIRAL: THE REALITY

In the same way that an upward energy spiral has a cumulative effect, a steadily growing negative energy spiral can often develop from fairly unspectacular beginnings. All it may take at the outset is a period of unmanaged stress. This could take the form of a severe viral illness such as a bad dose of 'flu from which you return to work before you've recovered. It might be a serious emotional trauma, such as a bereavement or the break-up of a relationship. It could be financial problems, or an unexpected change of job, increasing stress at work or a difficult pregnancy and demanding newborn, who struggles to establish a feeding and sleeping routine.

The consequences of all these situations can be dealt with if the appropriate action is taken to get yourself back on track, but if any of these should catch you at a low ebb, you may end up trapped in a pattern of negative coping strategies. These may take the form of a reliance on repeated shots of caffeine to get you through a tough day, and alcohol and/or sleeping tablets to help you unwind at night. If these are habitually combined with junk foods, eaten in a rush, instead of nutritious foods, eaten more slowly, you will be well on the way towards mental, emotional and physical exhaustion. When you reach this stage, your performance at work is likely to become pretty lacklustre, with poor levels of concentration and motivation, and your domestic life is also going to show signs of definite strain.

This can lead to a dizzying mixture of guilt, depression, resentment and anxiety – all profoundly energy-draining, negative emotions. If you take refuge in more alcohol, cigarettes and prescription drugs without examining the underlying problems through some form of talking therapy, the problems are almost guaranteed to worsen. By this point the motivation, energy and time-management skills that are needed to embark on a regular programme of physical fitness – even if it's only a brisk walk every day– are almost certainly going to be lacking.

If this negative situation continues long enough, you're likely to enter a phase of adrenal exhaustion or

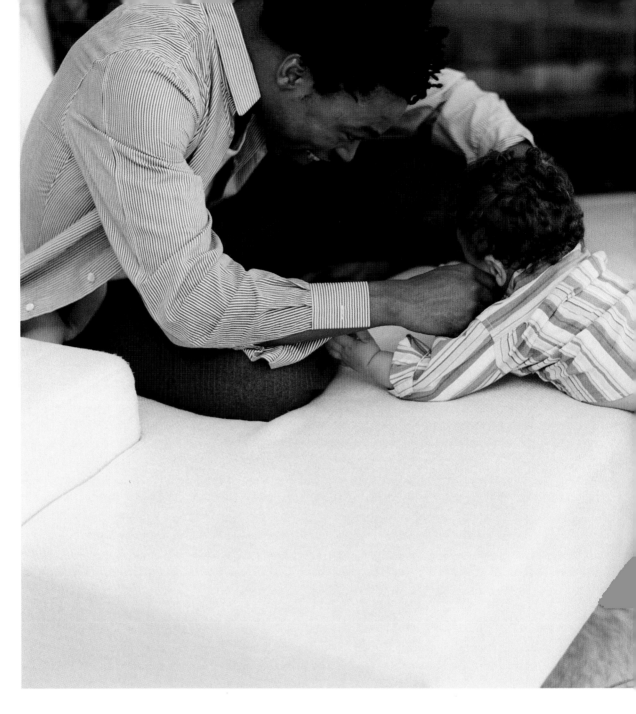

mental, emotional and physical burn-out. Once this has happened, it can have a noticeably adverse effect on your sleep patterns, your energy levels, the balance of your moods, digestive function, emotional responsiveness and your general ability to perform with mental sharpness. It is precisely at this point that a course of appropriate alternative or complementary medicine can be a life-saver.

Effective alternative treatment can be the vital catalyst you need to break the negative spiral. It may do no more at first than give you a safe space within which to express honestly how you feel about yourself and your situation. This in itself can be immensely therapeutic and self-revealing, but when these benefits are backed up with personalized prescriptions of alternative and complementary medicines, you should feel empowered to take small but steady steps towards improving your situation. A positive energy spiral is given the chance to emerge. And when you have put positive lifestyle changes in place, you may need only occasional support from your chosen alternative therapy.

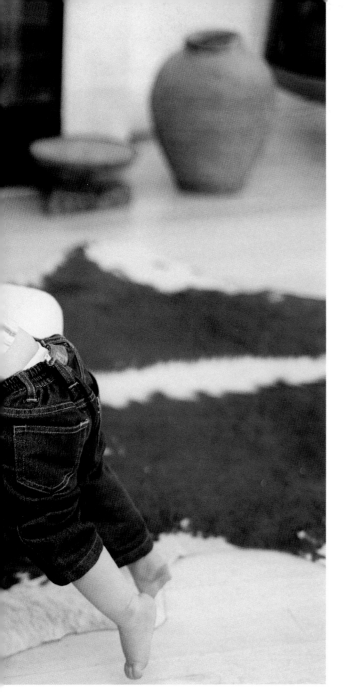

LEFT THERE ARE NO AGE RESTRICTIONS ON THE BENEFITS OF POSITIVE ENERGY. WHEN YOU FEEL EMOTIONALLY BALANCED AND PHYSICALLY AND MENTALLY ENERGIZED, LIFE IS FULL OF FUN AND SPARKLE – WHATEVER YOUR STAGE OF LIFE.

These patients will usually have come along for treatment having had all the relevant conventional medical tests done with all the results clear. When obvious conditions such as iron-deficiency anaemia, underactive thyroid function and glandular fever have been ruled out, the initial reaction is usually one of relief. A secondary feeling of dismay is, more often than not, rapidly sure to follow, as the patient who is tired all the time wonders just what the matter is. This can be quite an alarming worry to experience. When there is no obvious explanation for the symptoms of persistent tiredness, a real sense of anxiety can build up about what to do next. The reverse is true when you can find an explanation. Once the nature of the problem is diagnosed, the way is open for possible solutions to be explored and definite action to be taken.

If you're experiencing a general lack of sparkle and motivation that is of fairly recent onset, there's a very strong chance that adopting the measures outlined in this book will prove enough to kick-start your sense of vitality once again. More established problems with a low-level sense of fatigue may also be dealt with effectively by self-help. You can either take on board *Boost Your Energy Naturally* in its entirety or concentrate on your own 'vulnerable' areas (such as nutrition or physical fitness), which you know have been crying out for attention and are preventing you from reaching your energy potential.

On the other hand, when you move on to the next section – which is designed to help you to evaluate your basic level of mental, emotional and physical vitality – you may find that you have a well-established problem. Even if it turns out that you do suffer from a severe lack of energy on psychological and physical levels that refuse to respond to practical self-help measures, don't give up hope. The chances are that treatment from a professionally trained alternative or complementary practitioner will help you on your way to wellbeing.

THE AVERAGE SCENARIO: TIRED ALL THE TIME

For many of us, flagging energy levels are likely to be rather less dramatic than the scenario outlined above. Many of the patients I see regularly are nowhere near a state of complete burn-out, but they do realize that they aren't experiencing their optimum levels of mental, emotional and physical vitality either. People will often describe this state as a general sense of feeling unwell.

Identifying your current level of essential energy

Before you embark on your plan to boost your energy naturally, you need to identify the level it is at now. Answer the following questions, noting down the responses that apply to you.

How do you feel physically on waking?

A Refreshed and ready to start the day

B A bit slow to start, but fine once you're up and moving

C Muzzy-headed as if you need another three or four hours' sleep

How would you describe your sleep pattern?

A Generally sound and unbroken

B Pretty sound as a rule, but less refreshing after a stressful day

C Almost always fitful, with a propensity for waking up too early

How do you feel mentally on waking?

A Mentally and emotionally relaxed

B A bit tense, but fine once you're getting ready to start your day?

C Anxious and/or gloomy?

How much enthusiasm do you have for carrying out mental tasks during the day?

A More than enough

B On a good day plenty, but when the pressure builds it can show signs of flagging

C Very little, but somehow you get by

Do you tend to doze off if you have a quiet moment to yourself?

A Never

B Occasionally

C Frequently

BELOW WHEN YOU FEEL ENERGIZED AND EXHILARATED, YOU CAN FACE THE CURVES THAT LIFE THROWS YOU WITH ZEST.

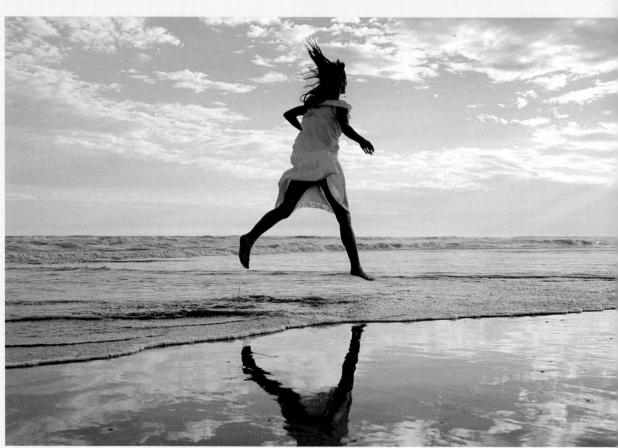

Do you rely on coffee, tea, caffeinated soft drinks and/or chocolate to help you keep up the pace?

A Hardly ever

B In small quantities and only when the pace heats up

C Every day

Do you depend on alcohol, drugs and/or cigarettes to help you unwind?

A Hardly ever

B Only under unusual circumstances and very infrequently

C Every day

Why do you eat?

A Because you feel genuinely hungry

B Sometimes from habit

C For comfort or because of boredom or sheer exhaustion

How do you react when you are offered an invitation for a night out?

A Do a quick mental calculation to check whether you're free, and respond with enthusiasm

B Wish you had an excuse, but go anyway and enjoy yourself

C Immediately say no even though you know you're free, because you don't feel up to it

How do you respond when faced with an unexpected challenge (a tight deadline, say, or an unexpected change in work plans or an off-the-cuff presentation)?

A Feel momentarily thrown, but quickly and effectively rise to the challenge

B Feel you'd rather get out of the situation, but cope well when you get into it

C Feel frozen and ineffective

How often do you suffer from colds and other minor infections?

A Once a year at most

B Twice a year or so

C Each one simply seems to run into another at a low-grade level

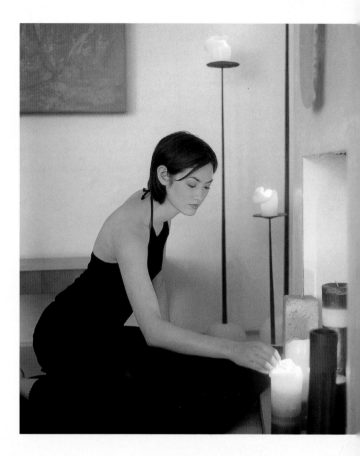

ABOVE **HEALTHY ENERGY LEVELS ARE ALL ABOUT BALANCE.**

How would you rate your sex drive?

A Enthusiastic and healthily balanced

B Generally okay, but with a tendency to nosedive when you are under too much pressure

C Flat as a pancake – most of the time you'd rather have a stiff drink

How often do you notice that the glands in your neck, armpits or groin feel swollen and tender?

A Never

B Only when you have a cold or 'flu

C Often

How often do you suffer from poor skin quality with a tendency to break out in spots, cold sores, unexplained rashes or boils?

A Never

B Only after a period of burning the candle at both ends

C Too often for comfort

If you scored mostly As

Congratulations! You really only need to read this book for interest's sake, as your all-round energy levels are extremely resilient and healthy. If there are any areas that you feel need an extra boost, you can probably get away with heading straight to the relevant chapters of this book. On the other hand, you're probably going to be the sort of person who is highly motivated and eager to explore any fresh ideas about maintaining your health, so you will no doubt read the entire book anyway.

If you scored mostly Bs

Your energy levels are generally okay, but may be subject to peaks and troughs in response to the amount of stress and pressure in your life at any given stage. It's worth taking action at this point in order to avoid the risk of descending into the negative energy spiral described on pages 15–16. The good news is that kick-starting your energy levels through the self-help measures outlined in this book should be straightforward and swift because you're starting from a reasonably healthy baseline. Don't worry – you don't have an uphill struggle in front of you.

If you scored mostly Cs

Don't despair, something can be done! Although you probably feel under par and unmotivated most of the time, the good news is that there are practical measures you can benefit from in order to take the first steps towards improved health and increased vitality. The trick is to start slowly and steadily, rather than being overwhelmed by taking a global view. In this situation it is undeniably best to start with a course of alternative treatment, rather than trying to make inroads into the problem through self-help measures alone. The time to back up the positive benefits of professional alternative medical help with appropriate changes in lifestyle is once a positive response has set in. But always remember that it's best to make small, cumulative changes rather than going for the short, sharp shock treatment. Taking things slowly will give you the chance to build on realistic foundations, which will ensure that your levels of vital energy can be transformed beyond your expectations.

BELOW EVERYONE HAS THE POTENTIAL TO BE BRIMMING WITH ENERGY AND WALKING WITH A SPRING IN THEIR STEP, NO MATTER HOW LOW THEIR CURRENT ENERGY LEVEL MAY BE.

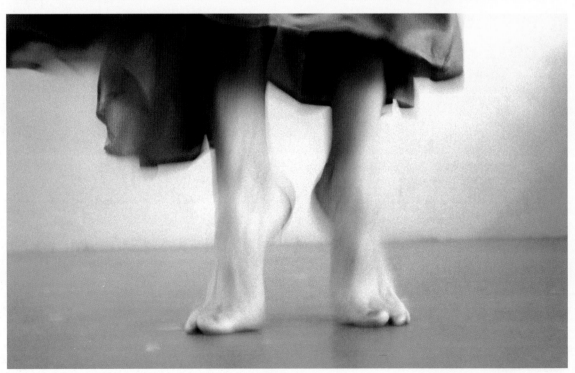

ENERGY MEDICINE: THE MAJOR SYSTEMS

This is not an exhaustive rundown of the systems of alternative medicine available. There are of course many more alternative and complementary therapies to choose from, but I regard the ones I have selected as the best-established and the most comprehensive systems of alternative healing available. Any of these would be an excellent choice if you are feeling burnt out and need an energy kick-start to get you moving on the right track.

ACUPUNCTURE

Acupuncture is an integral part of an approach to healing found in traditional Chinese medicine (which also includes Chinese herbal medicine and chi gong). It is an impressively long-established, very well road-tested system of alternative medicine – it has been suggested that the origins of acupuncture lie well beyond recorded history.

An acupuncturist works from the basic premise that optimum health is compromised when our flow of vital energy (called *chi*) becomes imbalanced. When this energy flows in a smooth and harmonious way, we should experience optimum mental, emotional and physical health. Should this smooth passage of healing energy become disrupted for any significant period of time, however, we are likely to start to experience symptoms that act as early warning signals that all is not well.

From the perspective of an acupuncturist, the most appropriate way to rectify this imbalance in vital energy is to insert ultra-fine needles into the surface of the skin at special points all over the body. The specific places where these needles need to be inserted will be determined by the symptoms experienced by each individual patient, as

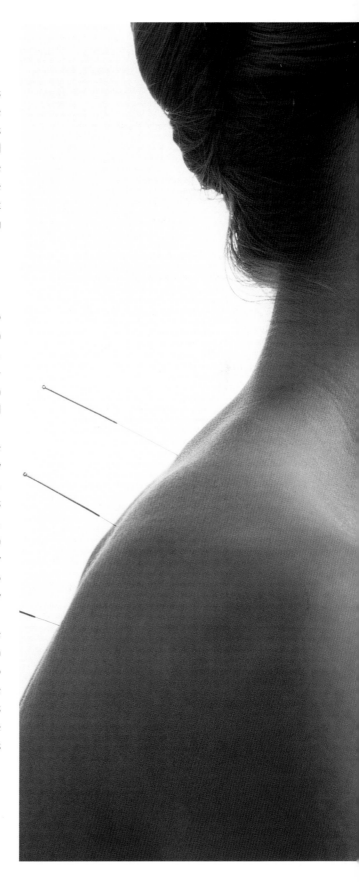

RIGHT **THE EARLIEST ACUPUNCTURE NEEDLES ARE THOUGHT TO HAVE BEEN MADE FROM SILVER, COPPER, BAMBOO OR GOLD. TODAY THE EXTRA-FINE NEEDLES USED BY THE AVERAGE ACUPUNCTURIST ARE MADE FROM STAINLESS STEEL WITH COPPER TIPS.**

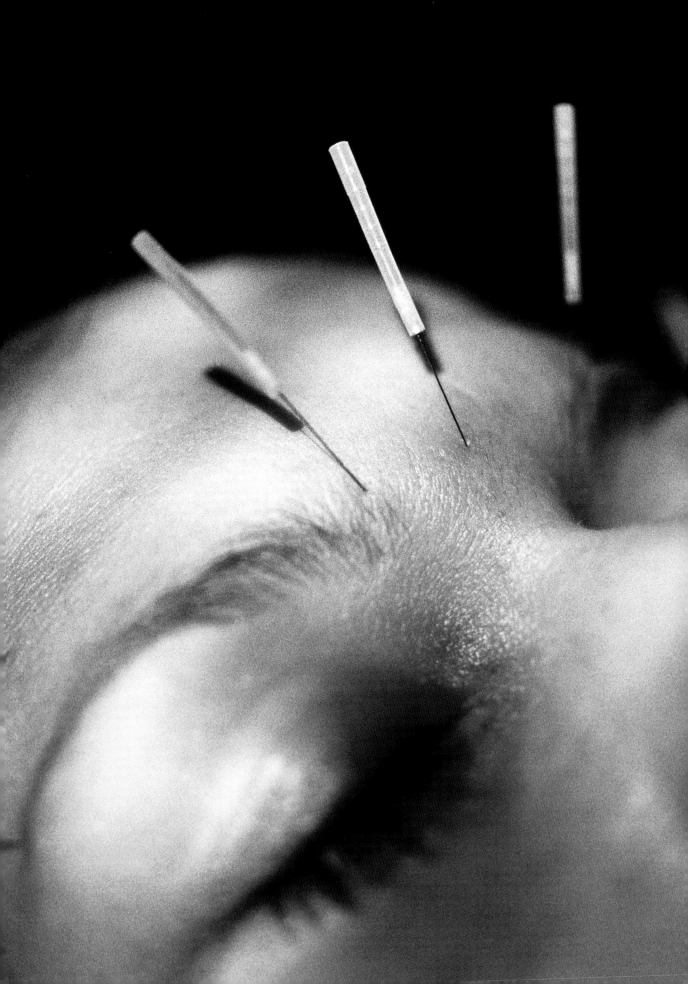

acupuncture, in common with other types of holistic therapies, places great emphasis on the need to treat each patient as unique.

If you have consulted an acupuncturist, you may well be familiar with the charts of the body that trace the location and pathways of meridians. These are the invisible tracks that are thought to be arranged in a continuous loop of major and subsidiary pathways covering the entire body. There are approximately 35 of these channels in total, with the main tracks radiating along the surface of the arms, legs, torso and head.

The meridians play a vitally important role in acupuncture, as they are the channels along which *chi* is thought to flow. As a result, inserting acupuncture needles at appropriate points along these tracks (it has been estimated that there are a total of 365 traditional acupuncture points lying on the meridians that form connections with the major organs) appears to activate the body's own healing potential. And thus we are back with the basic concept of stimulating vital healing energy.

The Consultation

Acupuncturists rely a great deal on observation when they are taking information about a patient's medical history. Detailed examination of the tongue and pulse is crucial, as any imbalances in the body as a whole may be revealed through irregularities in the colour or texture of the tongue or by a weak or rapid pulse.

Once a detailed history has been recorded and a general diagnosis made, the practitioner will set to work, inserting a chosen number of acupuncture needles into appropriate points on the body. This is not as alarming as it sounds. After an initial sensation of mild awareness on the insertion of each acupuncture needle, there shouldn't be any further discomfort. The needles may be left in position for up to 30 minutes, with the practitioner deciding which points need to be slightly rotated in order to have an extra stimulating effect on the flow of energy.

LEFT **ACUPUNCTURE IS THOUGHT TO WORK BY STIMULATING THE BALANCED FLOW OF ENERGY THROUGHOUT THE BODY.**

Sensations during treatment will vary depending on your individual response, but commonly reported feelings include a slight tingling or warmth that runs along the meridian being treated. Once a session is over and the needles are removed, you shouldn't experience any pain or bleeding. To gain the most from the therapy, it's often a good idea to avoid any activity that may put a strain on your body for a couple of hours or so after treatment. This is one occasion when going for a swim or a run is not advisable, nor is having a heavy meal.

As acupuncture is very much a holistic therapy that aims to rectify imbalances in the body as a whole, you're also very likely to be given advice on changes in lifestyle that will help to maximize and support the benefits of treatment. These will be tailored to meet your individual needs, and may include dietary adjustments, taking up gentle exercise and relaxation techniques. If this broad approach is successful, it should have a significant effect on balancing your energy levels, promoting healthy reserves of vitality during the day and enabling you to relax at night.

What can acupuncture treat?

In common with other alternative therapies, acupuncture treats the person as a whole, rather than the condition, but it is helpful to know the impressive number of health problems that have been found to respond well to this therapy. They include the following:

- **Recurrent infections (cystitis, colds, sinusitis, etc.)**
- **Unexplained fatigue**
- **Lowered libido**
- **Allergies (rhinitis or hay fever)**
- **Anxiety**
- **Back pain**
- **Depression**
- **Skin complaints (including eczema and psoriasis)**
- **Tension headaches**
- **Migraines**
- **Sleep problems**

AYURVEDA

Ayurveda is a holistic health system that has been practised for hundreds of years in India and Sri Lanka, and is now starting to become increasingly popular in the West. This is due partly to the general upsurge in interest in alternative therapies that we have seen during the past two decades, and partly to the popularization of ayurvedic principles of healing through the work of well-known practitioners such as Deepak Chopra and Bharti Vyas.

From an ayurvedic perspective, each of us has a basic mental, emotional and physical constitution that is made up of a combination of three basic *doshas* called *vata*, *pitta* and *kapha*. And guess what? The word dosha is a term that yet again can be roughly translated to mean vital energy. When our doshas are in healthy balance, we should experience good health and balanced mental, emotional and physical energy. On the other hand, if they become imbalanced for any significant period of time, this basic disharmony is likely to manifest itself in the symptoms of ill health.

Ayurvedic practitioners believe that the fundamental balance of the doshas in each person is established in the womb, depending on the inherited characteristics that each of us is given by our birth parents at the moment of conception. This is our basic physical and mental constitution. This need not be regarded as being graven in stone, however, as other influences can have a significant impact on the balance of our individual doshas. The quality of the diet that we enjoy regularly, the amount and kind of exercise we take and our ability to manage excessive stress effectively all impact on our doshas. If we make wise choices, we can maximize the strengths in our basic constitution, while ministering to the more vulnerable areas.

Unfortunately, the reverse also holds true. An excess of negative mental, emotional and physical influences can eventually grind down even a generally tough and resilient constitution.

It is helpful to bear in mind that the balance in each constitution between the doshas is essentially fluid and dynamic in nature and as result is subject to frequent fluctuation, depending on the environmental factors that are operating on us at any given time.

A Quick Tour of the Three Doshas

For an ayurvedic practitioner, the balance between the three doshas described below is of fundamental importance, as the doshas are seen as supporting all of the vital processes that affect our mental, emotional and physical health. As a result, this balance within our bodies has an influence on everything from our physical characteristics (including body shape, ability to fight infection and underlying patterns of energy) to our individual personality traits.

The Vata Profile

The main features of the vata dosha can be summed up as fidgety and changeable.

Pattern of energy Characterized by bursts of extremely high vitality that can suddenly plummet, or 'crash and burn'.

Mental and emotional features Include a remarkable capacity for creativity, with a proportional tendency to become quickly distracted by new ideas. When

LEFT VATA TYPES CAN BE VERY CREATIVE IN GOOD HEALTH.

enthusiasm is present, it is there in bucketloads. Nervous exhaustion is a constant danger in this constitutional type.

Physical features Include a slim build with a tendency to long bones and an elongated facial shape.

Common symptoms or indicators

- Erratic, constantly fluctuating levels of emotional, mental and physical energy
- Anxiety and insecurity
- Poor long-term memory and general inability to focus on the task in hand
- Poor-quality, fitful sleep
- Unstable libido as a result of hugely fluctuating energy levels
- Constipation and other problems related to low-grade dehydration such as headaches and dry skin

Aggravating factors

- Lack of good-quality, regular sleep
- Extended mental and emotional stress
- Suppression of anxiety and worry
- Over-reliance on junk foods and alcohol
- Lack of structure and routine
- Lack of regular, 'grounding' exercise or system of movement such as yoga
- Erratic eating patterns
- Excessive use of stimulants in an effort to keep up the pace (e.g. coffee and caffeinated soft drinks)
- Neglecting to moisturize and care for the skin
- Change of season from summer to autumn and winter

The Kapha Profile

This dosha can be summed up as solid, sturdy and steady.

Pattern of energy Slow with an underlying tendency to feel lethargic and sleepy.

Mental and emotional features A notable propensity for reliability and

emotional stability. When this dosha is in optimum balance, it leads to a strongly nurturing, caring nature with a great capacity for calmness and contentment. The downside of this make-up is a risk of mental and emotional sluggishness, including a resistance to embracing new challenges or opportunities.

Physical features Include a proneness towards a slow metabolism with a corresponding tendency to gain weight easily. The skin of someone with a kapha constitution may look oily and feel cold to the touch.

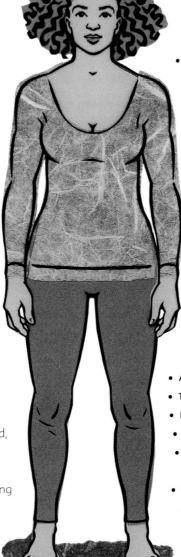

Common symptoms or indicators

- Lack of flexibility
- Lack of drive
- Intolerance of being rushed or pushed into anything
- Obstinacy
- Constant chilliness
- Low libido with slow sexual arousal
- Sluggish digestion with an ongoing problem with indigestion and/or constipation

Aggravating factors

- Boredom and lack of stimulation
- Blows to self-esteem and confidence (e.g. relationship break-up or loss of job)
- Becoming socially withdrawn
- Overeating in search of comfort or distraction
- A sedentary lifestyle
- Too much sleep
- Becoming chilled
- Taking sleeping pills or tranquillizers
- An excess of fatty foods (dairy or fried items), sweets or red meat
- Change of season to midwinter or spring

LEFT **KAPHA TYPES ARE OFTEN EXTREMELY SINGLE-MINDED.**

The Pitta Profile

The primary characteristics of the pitta dosha are tendencies to be fiery and passionate.

Pattern of energy In good health when this dosha is in optimum balance the result is an extremely focused, energetic person who is able to achieve an enormous amount through sheer force of will.

Mental and emotional features Include terrific confidence, enthusiasm and ambition. Memory is likely to be sharp, with a striking ability to assimilate information quickly and accurately.

Physical features Include fair, sensitive skin that can burn quickly and easily, with a tendency to freckle and 'break out' into rashes. The body shape is likely to be well proportioned.

Common symptoms

- Despite such enormous, sustained energy reserves, there's a major risk of complete burn-out if stress triggers remain out of control for too long
- Emotional 'shortfuse' with marked irritability and fiery anger. This can lead to hasty, unwise decisions being made
- A tendency to perspire quickly and profusely when under pressure
- Stress-related diarrhoea

Aggravating factors

- Repressed anger
- Becoming mentally, emotionally and physically exhausted
- Becoming physically overheated
- Erratic eating patterns
- Eating too much red meat or highly spiced, salty foods
- Repeated courses of antibiotics
- Change of season from spring to summer

Achieving and Maintaining Essential Balance

You should always bear in mind that, from an ayurvedic perspective, the three doshas are likely to be present in each of us to at least some degree at any given time. This is why many of us will probably recognize some elements from each of the three doshas in ourselves. When you are in a state of optimum health, these characteristics should balance each other out.

On the other hand, when you become rundown and stressed out, you may be conscious that the negative features of one dosha, or a combination of two, come to the fore. This is when action needs to be taken in order to establish healthy balance once again.

An excellent initial step for action is to study the lists of factors that can be responsible for triggering an excess amount of each dosha. For example, if you are aware that you tend to become dominant in kapha when under stress, it makes sense to cut right down on fatty foods, take up stimulating exercise and get out and about more. If you exhibit a combination of pitta and vata dominance when the pressure intensifies, you need to set in train some lifestyle changes that will make you feel calmer and more 'grounded', and help you to make the most of your energy potential.

Always remember to use this information as creatively and as loosely as you wish. Rather than fretting about not fitting neatly into

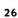

LEFT **PITTA TYPES ARE OUTGOING, SOCIABLE AND PASSIONATE BY NATURE.**

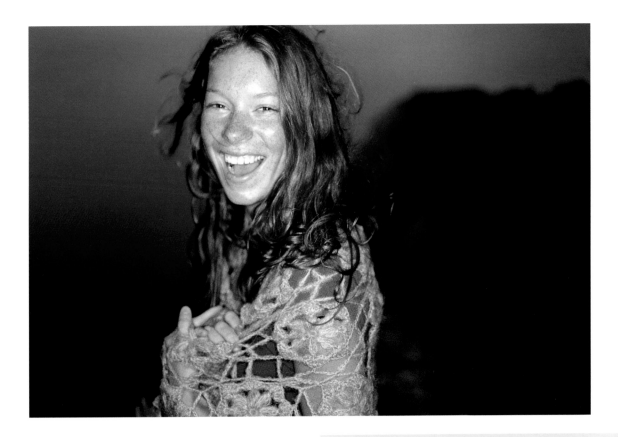

ABOVE **BALANCED DOSHAS MEAN BALANCED ENERGY LEVELS.**

a specific dosha type when things do go out of balance, use this information as a fresh perspective on understanding the way that mental, emotional and physical energy levels can ebb and flow in the body.

The Consultation

It is well worth considering treatment from a properly qualified ayurvedic practitioner. Just like traditional Chinese practitioners, ayurvedic physicians are likely to carry out a thorough physical examination when you consult them for the first time. Treatment will often take the form of a prescription of herbal medicines, advice on dietary changes, regular exercise, massage, relaxation techniques or steam treatments. Once again, this is an approach to healing that is very much concerned with stimulating optimum health on physical, mental and emotional levels. For examples of conditions that respond well to this therapy, see the lists of symptoms given under each dosha heading or the box on the right.

What can ayurveda treat?

Ayurveda is another holistic therapy that looks at the whole person rather than homing in on treating merely the symptoms of an illness. In fact, you do not even need to be ill before consulting an ayurvedic practitioner because of its potential as a true preventative system of health care. Ayurveda can treat a number of chronic conditions, including:

- **Skin conditions (e.g. psoriasis and eczema)**
- **Sleep problems**
- **Digestive disorders**
- **General stress-related problems**
- **Anxiety and depression**
- **Premenstrual syndrome**
- **Migraine**
- **Arthritis**
- **Asthma and bronchitis**
- **Cystitis**
- **Hay fever**

HOMEOPATHY

One of the most popular and thoroughly road-tested alternative therapies available to us is homeopathy. Practised across the globe for the past 200 years or so, this system is based on the principle of like curing like, and remedies come in the form of tiny pills. It can be used practically on a self-help basis to treat a range of minor ailments from stomach upsets and sprains to physical and emotional shock. In the hands of a properly trained practitioner it can be employed to treat an impressive range of chronic conditions effectively. In addition, it is one of the most appropriate therapies to consider on a preventative basis if you feel that you have not yet reached the stage of definable illness, but know that your self-healing energy reserves are in need of a boost.

There are no age barriers to treatment, and, providing there is no mechanical obstacle standing in the way of improvement (e.g. a misaligned disc in the spine, or tissue that has been irreversibly changed), there should always be some degree of improvement after treatment. See the box on page 31 for some of the conditions for which homeopathy is suitable.

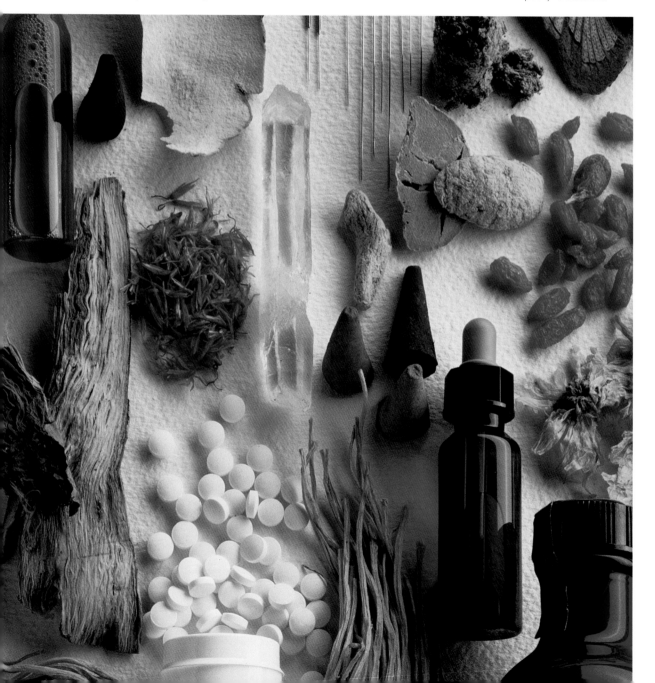

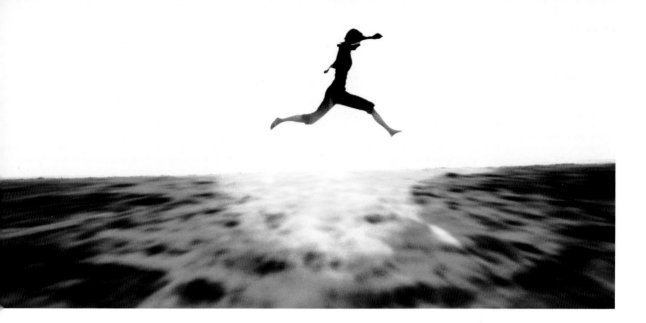

The Consultation

The first thing that is noticeable about the initial homeopathic consultation is its length: it should take between and 60 and 90 minutes. During this time, the homeopath will form a detailed picture of your experience of health right across the board. As a result, some of the questions that you are asked may be surprising in their depth and detail – especially if you're used to the average eight-minute consultation at your doctor's practice.

Once all this information has been gathered, the homeopath will try to match your symptoms to the choice of the most appropriate homeopathic remedy (which may be made from one of a range of substances including plant, mineral or herbal ingredients). If the choice of remedy is effective, not only should any symptoms of ill health improve, but there should be a perceptible increase in emotional, mental and physical energy as well. Homeopathic patients are often delighted by how their overall sense of wellbeing increases, in proportion to the improvement in their eczema, tension headaches, recurrent infections or asthma.

Whatever homeopathic remedy is selected can be given in a wide range of forms, including tablets,

granules, powders, liquids or wafers. If it is a very high-potency (strength) remedy, it is not uncommon to take just one dose then wait for a week or so to assess the response. On the other hand, some of the liquid remedies can be taken daily. The practitioner will evaluate the vitality of each patient and work at an appropriate level with it.

Some Basic Homeopathic Energy Profiles

Homeopaths will often talk about constitutional pictures, which in many ways we can regard as being similar to the ayurvedic doshas outlined on pages 24–6. In other words, each of us is born with a number of constitutional characteristics that influence the amount of energy we enjoy, our mental and emotional health, our physical attributes, and our overall ability to fight off illness. Our constitutional picture is likely to fluctuate with our age, lifestyle and whatever pressures are operating on us at any given stage of our life. However, you may already have noticed that certain patterns of psychological and physical imbalance tend to come to the fore when the going has been too tough for too long.

In truth, more than 20 constitutional types could be described in the next few pages, but there is simply not enough space to cover these within this book. I've chosen to explore three major homeopathic energy types that most closely complement the ayurvedic doshas of vata, kapha and pitta.

ABOVE **SUCCESSFUL HOMEOPATHIC TREATMENT CAN MEAN A SURGE OF WELLBEING FOR SOME PATIENTS.**
LEFT **COMPLEMENTARY REMEDIES PRODUCED FROM NATURAL SUBSTANCES PROVIDE A VERSATILE APPROACH TO HEALTH.**

The Phosphorus Profile

This profile can be best summed up as energetic, outgoing and sensitive. Owing to their extrovert, sociable nature, phosphorus types respond especially negatively to feelings of loneliness and isolation, rendering them susceptible to becoming emotionally depressed and physically rundown.

Pattern of energy Volatile, moving from very high mental, emotional and physical energy at one moment, to complete exhaustion the next. Evening can be an especially vulnerable time for phosphorus types, when energy levels can drain away without much warning.

Mental and emotional features Include acute sensitivity and empathy with other people's feelings, almost to the point of being psychic. Phosphorus types often pick up on other people's moods without consciously realizing it – another reason why they can become emotionally drained very quickly.

Physical features Include slenderness with fine, long bones. Hair is often fine, too, while with eyes are large with very long lashes.

Common symptoms

- Anxiety
- Mental and emotional hypersensitivity (especially when alone)
- Unexplained fatigue
- Weakness of the throat leading to recurrent throat infections and tonsillitis
- Chest infections, bronchitis or asthma
- A tendency to nosebleeds or easy bruising
- Kidney and bladder infections

Aggravating factors

- A growth spurt
- Excessive physical effort
- Changes in atmospheric pressure (e.g. before a thunderstorm)
- A diet too high in salt
- Loss of body fluids (e.g. heavy perspiration or after a menstrual period)

The Nux Vomica Profile

Keynote aspects of this homeopathic profile are being mentally, emotionally and physically driven, with the corresponding tendency to become overwrought and to operate on a short fuse.

Pattern of energy Can be astonishingly high when focused on achieving a specific goal. Morning is almost always a low point, with energy levels rising steadily throughout the day.

Mental and emotional features Include enormous capacity to absorb information under pressure, with a proportionate ability to work to punishing deadlines. Common features include a quick temper and easily triggered irritability. If life in the fast lane goes on for too long, mental and emotional burn-out can set in.

Physical features Often include a spare, slim build resulting from a fast metabolism, pushing hard to do competitive exercise regularly and eating irregularly. On the other hand, the opposite picture can emerge in hard-pressed executives who live on junk food, drink large amounts of alcohol regularly, take no exercise and drive everywhere. As a result, they become out of shape and overweight.

Common symptoms

- Inability to relax
- Drowsiness
- Extreme impatience and irritability
- Insomnia
- Indigestion, lack of appetite and persistent constipation
- Tension headaches and migraines
- Exhausted and 'hung over' on waking

Aggravating factors

- Too much mental, emotional and physical pressure over an extended period
- Repressed resentment and anger
- Reliance on alcohol, cigarettes and sleeping pills to unwind
- Excessive amounts of coffee and other stimulants to keep up with the pace
- Too much junk food in the diet
- Sleep deprivation

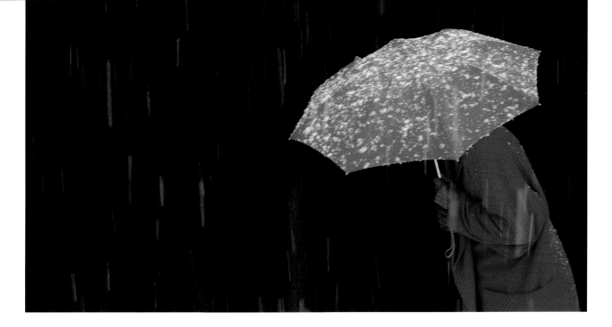

The Calc Carb Profile

The main features of this profile are sluggishness, slowness and chilliness.

Pattern of energy Persistently low, with even the smallest effort triggering a sense of extreme mental and physical exhaustion.

Mental and emotional features Include constant anxiety that is related to an extreme lack of self-confidence and self-esteem. When life is in balance, this remedy profile can be methodical, emotionally stable and reliable; however, when things go off track sluggishness and lack of motivation set in.

Physical features Include a marked tendency to gain weight easily, as a result of a sluggish metabolism (thyroid function can often be a problem) combined with a definite pattern of comfort eating and lack of exercise. Skin is likely to be pale, oily and chilly.

Common symptoms

- Lack of motivation
- Anxiety
- Depression
- Recurrent infections (colds, chest infections, ear infections and sinusitis)
- Poor bone density (osteoporosis and poor-quality teeth)
- Slow digestion leading to indigestion
- Constipation
- Migraine

ABOVE **WEATHER CONDITIONS CAN HAVE AN IMPACT ON YOUR HEALTH, WITH SOME SYMPTOMS BEING MARKEDLY MORE SEVERE IN DAMP, COLD WEATHER.**

Aggravating factors

- Emotional stress and pressure
- Physical effort (e.g. taking up vigorous exercise too quickly)
- Comfort eating (especially if it includes stodgy, sweet or fatty foods)
- Boredom and lack of stimulation
- Becoming chilled and damp

What can homeopathy treat?

Common problems that can be treated with homeopathy include:

- **Persistent fatigue**
- **Recurrent infections**
- **Tension headaches and migraine**
- **Eczema and psoriasis**
- **Asthma**
- **Hay fever**
- **Premenstrual syndrome**
- **Arthritis**
- **Irritable bowel syndrome**
- **Anxiety and depression**
- **Lowered libido**

PUTTING IT ALL TOGETHER

By now, certain recurring patterns should have started to become obvious in the profiles sketched previously. Ideally, you will recognize some of your own patterns of energy in these. But don't worry if you can't. This in no way means that the advice outlined in the rest of the book is not for you. On the contrary, it simply means that you can apply its principles more generally.

On the other hand, if you find that you recognize yourself in any of the profiles – vata/phosphorus, pitta/nux vomica or kapha/calc carb, you will obviously benefit more from the specific advice offered for these particular profiles. Please bear in mind that these descriptions are very generalized in order to create as broad a picture as possible.

In order to draw this information even more closely together, you need to explore briefly how your mental, emotional and physical energy levels are likely to ebb and flow naturally during an average day. This will give you a very useful picture of how energy in action can affect you in different ways, depending on the sort of basic constitution that you have. The point of this exercise is also to impart some initial, sensible advice on how to begin to apply some of the basic principles of boosting your energy naturally. After all, we all have to start somewhere.

The Early Evening Slump

This situation can apply to the vata/phosphorus energy type – in other words, to those of us who may be slightly slow to get started in the mornings, but who generally cope well enough as the day gets under way. However, you may be dismayed to find that, once you return home at the end of a working day, you suddenly feel as though someone has switched off your energy supply at its source. If this pattern sounds all too familiar, the following advice is worth adopting to try to break this negative energy cycle and banish it to being a thing of the past:

- This constitutional type has a general tendency to feel exhausted as a result of low blood sugar levels or low-

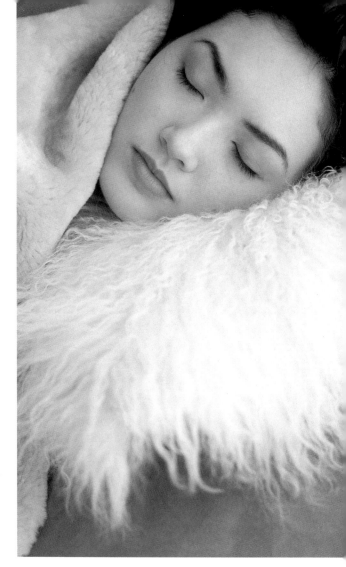

ABOVE **SOUND, RESTFUL SLEEP IS THE FOUNDATION OF VIBRANT HEALTH FOR EVERYBODY.**

grade dehydration. You need to make a point during the day of eating something small but nutritious every couple of hours, and always make sure that you drink six large glasses of water a day. If this seems difficult to achieve at work, make a habit of keeping a large bottle of still mineral water and a glass on your desk.

- Always avoid the temptation to collapse in front of the television with a snack and a stiff drink, as this is almost certainly going to aggravate the problem.

- During the lighter spring and summer nights, take a short walk in the fresh air before your evening meal. Breathing in some fresh air at this point in the day can go a long way towards preventing physical and mental exhaustion later.

- During the darker winter nights, opt instead for doing 15 or 20 minutes of yoga at home, guided by a book or some of the excellent home videos available. This should neatly circumvent the problem of lack of motivation that can understandably hold us back from venturing out to a class on a cold, dark, wet winter's night.

- If you need an energy boost to perk you up in preparation for a night out, treat yourself to a revitalizing shower using a shower gel that is infused with citrus essential oils. If, on the other hand, you're staying in and want a more leisurely experience, soak in a vitality-inducing bath. Ensure that the water is warm rather than overly hot, as this can make you feel enervated, rather than stimulated.

BELOW **WATER CAN BE EITHER INVIGORATING OR RELAXING DEPENDING ON YOUR NEEDS AT THE TIME.**

The Early Morning Slump

This energy pattern is readily recognizable, as waking up can be a vulnerable period for pitta/nux vomica energy types (morning is a time usually associated with vata/phosphorus types). As a result, peace and quiet at this time is an absolute necessity. Otherwise anyone unfortunate enough to be around you is likely to have his or her head bitten off. As the day progresses, things steadily improve, with your mental, emotional and physical energy levels reaching their peak by the end of the day. This can set up an instinctive, negative pattern of working later and later into the early hours of the following day, making it consistently harder for you to drag yourself out of bed when the alarm goes off. Try the following initial steps in an attempt to break this negative cycle:

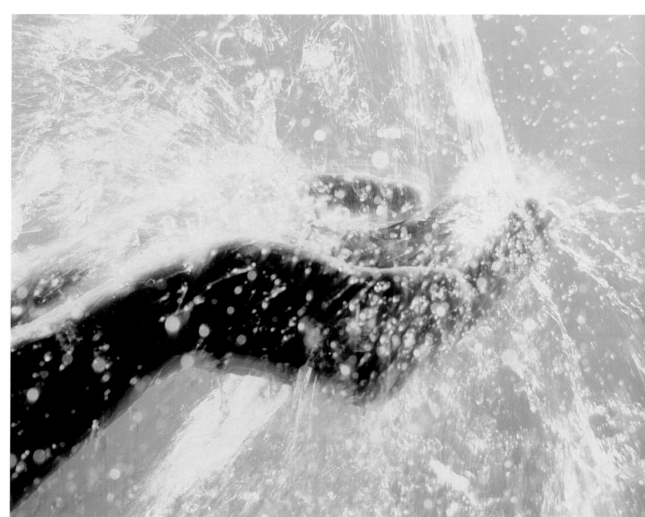

- It may be stating the obvious, but it's absolutely vital to ensure that you maintain a regular routine of sound sleep if you want to avoid feeling grumpy and overtired when you wake up in the morning. However unnatural it may feel at first – and there is no doubt that you will want to rebel against this regime at the outset – make a point of going to sleep regularly before midnight at the latest. Once you become used to this new sleep pattern, you will gradually discover that your mind and body become programmed for rest more easily.

- Use simple, practical alternative measures to help induce a feeling of relaxation and drowsiness once you are in bed. Listen to a favourite piece of soothing music; if you prefer to be read to sleep, listen to a talking book. You could also try sipping a warm mug of calming camomile tea, or put a drop or two of slumber-inducing lavender essential oil on your pillow to encourage restful sleep.

- As instituting this new regime is likely to be traumatic, cut yourself some slack, and be ruthless about giving yourself enough time to get organized in the morning. You may feel as if you are going against the grain at first, but begin a habit of getting up 15 minutes earlier than is strictly necessary. Giving yourself this precious interval of extra time can effectively sidestep your feeling pressured and fraught at a time when you know you're going to feel particularly fragile. How you choose to use this additional window of opportunity is entirely up to you and your individual preference. Taking the time to have breakfast rather than grabbing a cup of coffee and a slice of toast as you run out the door, enjoying a long shower, meditating or just sitting and gathering your thoughts can all be ways of consciously preparing for the day ahead.

- Always avoid relying on sleeping tablets to try to switch off after working late. Sleeping tablets can cause their own extra problems when used frequently, and they're almost certainly going to contribute towards you feeling 'hung over' on waking and drowsy during the first part of your day. If additional help is needed to establish a healthier, regular pattern of sleep, opt instead for less addictive herbal sedative preparations. These should help you to unwind without the problems associated with conventional sleeping tablets.

- Resist the temptation to doze off during the day, as this can make you feel disoriented, depressed and moody, rather than invigorated. If you sleep for any substantial time during the day, it can also make it that bit harder to drop off easily to sleep at night.

BELOW VAPORIZING AROMATHERAPY OILS IS A PLEASURABLE WAY OF CREATING A MOOD-BALANCING ATMOSPHERE. BELOW LEFT LAVENDER HAS RELAXING AND MEDICINAL PROPERTIES THAT CAN BOOST YOUR SENSE OF WELLBEING.

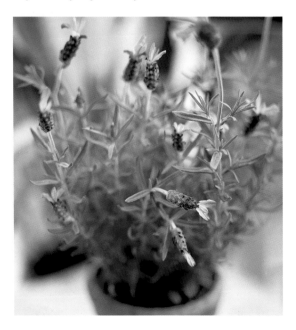

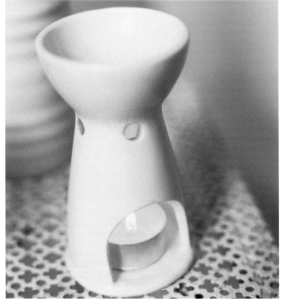

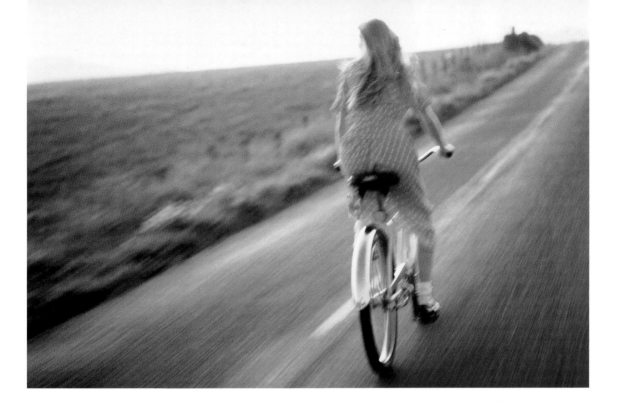

Constantly Exhausted

Rather than having a specific vulnerable spot during the day when energy levels are obviously flagging, kapha/calc carb energy types can be susceptible to feelings of persistent fatigue and drowsiness at any time of day. If you recognize this tendency within yourself, you need to give priority to basic, practical measures that will present you with the best chance of enjoying a steady flow of vitality throughout the day. Within the context of this energy picture, stimulation is the key to energy boosting, rather than rest and replenishment.

- This constitutional profile thrives on healthy amounts of mental, emotional and physical stimulation. Hence it's important to avoid slipping into lifestyle habits that create an undemanding tempo. One of the best ways of avoiding this is to monitor the amount of sleep that is had every night. While the other two constitutional types need to make sure that plenty of good-quality rest is taken, kapha/calc carb types should be vigilant that they're not slipping over into a pattern of getting too much sleep. As a general rule, it's best to try to get to sleep before midnight, making sure to rise after seven hours of good-quality, solid sleep. Extending into ten or more hours regularly is likely to have a soporific rather than stimulating effect.

ABOVE **CYCLING IS AN EXCELLENT FORM OF AEROBIC EXERCISE, WHICH IS ESPECIALLY BENEFICIAL IF YOU ALWAYS FEEL EXHAUSTED WITH DEPLETED ENERGY LEVELS.**

- If you feel that you have a generally sluggish constitution and you're employed in a sedentary job, make it an absolute priority to take up a stimulating form of exercise that conditions your heart and lungs, and generally gets the circulation moving. In this situation expending energy brings fantastic returns by boosting vitality. If you take up a form of exercise that involves being out and about in the open air, you're likely to find it brings extra benefits in the form of sleeping more readily and deeply at night.

- Avoid the temptation to 'graze' constantly throughout the day, or to eat extra-large meals for comfort or because you are bored. Either of these patterns of eating will be likely to make you feel the opposite of energized: you're far more likely to find that you feel drowsy or uncomfortably bloated, or perhaps both.

- Start the day with a stimulating burst of citrus-scented essential oils. One way to do this is to vaporize the oil in a custom-made essential-oil burner as you are preparing to start your day. An alternative is to use an invigorating shower gel, which can be applied to damp skin with a bath mitt and lathered up to give a refreshing shower.

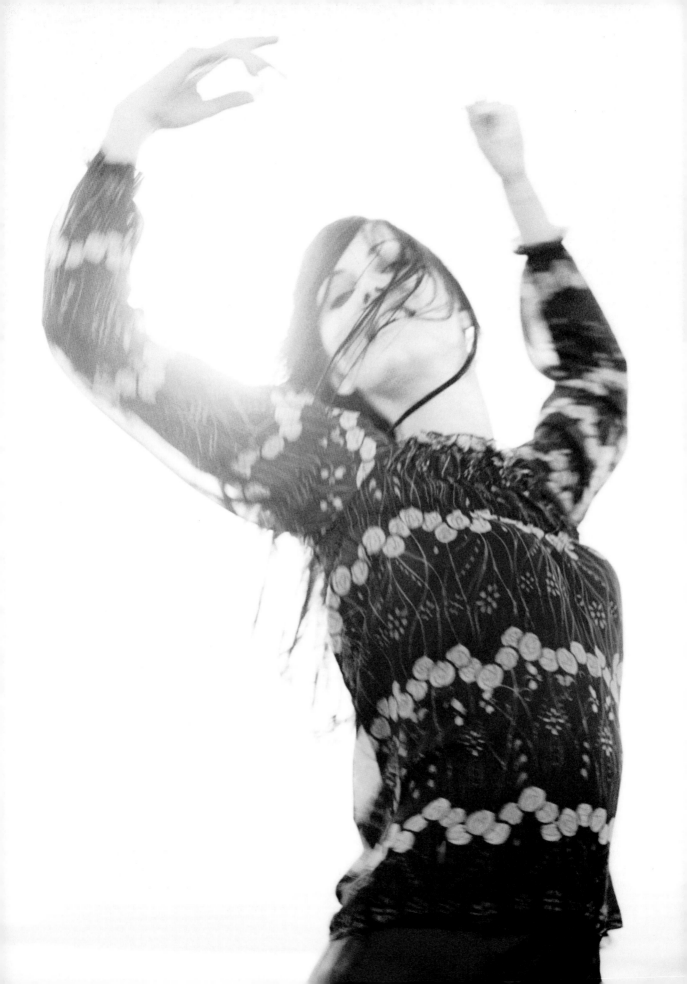

2 First steps

Before you learn how to set about stimulating your baseline levels of all-round vitality, it makes a great deal of sense to spend a little time exploring any hidden aspects of your lifestyle that may be draining your energy. Simply taking trouble to identify what these are will mean that you make a flying start. The sooner these negative aspects are effectively dealt with, the more rapidly any additional energy-boosting measures you adopt will have a much more noticeable impact. It's basically a question of removing any obstacles that may be standing in your way so that you are free to move forwards.

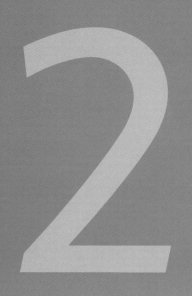

Kicking out the negative

Common energy drainers

It is easy to drain your energy without being conscious of doing so. Recognizing and acknowledging the common energy drainers in your attitude and lifestyle is the first step towards getting these negative aspects out of your system.

- **Instinctive negative thought patterns and responses (e.g. lack of motivation, fear of change, pessimism and inertia)**
- **Disturbed sleep pattern**
- **Reliance on adrenaline 'rushes' to keep you moving and motivated**
- **Poorly managed stress**
- **Negative self-image and low self-confidence**
- **Lack of exercise**
- **Loneliness**
- **Depression**

OPPOSITE **DANCING IS AN ENJOYABLE WAY OF EXPRESSING YOUR FEELINGS AS WELL AS CONDITIONING YOUR BODY.** LEFT **DEPRESSION CAN MAKE YOU FEEL CONTINUALLY DEPLETED AND EXHAUSTED.**

ACCENTUATING THE POSITIVE: PUTTING BASIC ENERGY FOUNDATIONS IN PLACE

If you recognize that one or more of the following energy drainers applies to you, it's time to take action using the practical strategies recommended below. Above all, don't put this off. Take action today, and you may be amazed at the results.

Combating Negative Thought Patterns

Lack of Motivation

You need to take a hard look at what's holding you back from feeling enthusiastic about tasks at hand: is it boredom or fear of being overwhelmed, or are you genuinely unsuited to what you are trying to do in either your personal or professional life?

Boredom always needs to be tackled, as it's one of the most draining states we can experience. If you feel stuck in a professional or personal rut, you need to make a deliberate point of shaking things up by introducing yourself to new challenges. Just make sure that these challenges are realistic and within your abilities, so that the end result will be confidence-boosting, encouraging you to move further along this positive learning curve.

Deliberately change any routines that may have become stifling rather than productive, however small these initial changes may necessarily need to be. The main thing is to avoid the sensation of being blocked or boxed in. After all, nothing is quite so inhibiting and demotivating as feeling that you can't take any positive action.

Fear of being out of your depth also needs evaluating in order to work out if this is well-founded or you are in fact unconsciously using it as an avoidance technique so that you can duck out of challenging situations. When you're faced with a situation from which you instinctively want to back away, it helps to stop for a moment and consider how sound this reaction is. Ideally, you need to try to stand back from your initial response and picture yourself coping well with whatever challenge has presented itself.

If, on reflection, you decide you could actually deal effectively with it, it's worth taking the plunge and having a go. On the other hand, if you genuinely think that you can't do justice to it, you can say no, then evaluate the next situation that comes along. The main thing is experiencing the liberating feeling that comes with having made a considered decision, rather than being slave to a knee-jerk reaction. This approach helps you to feel that you are more in control of choices you need to make in your life.

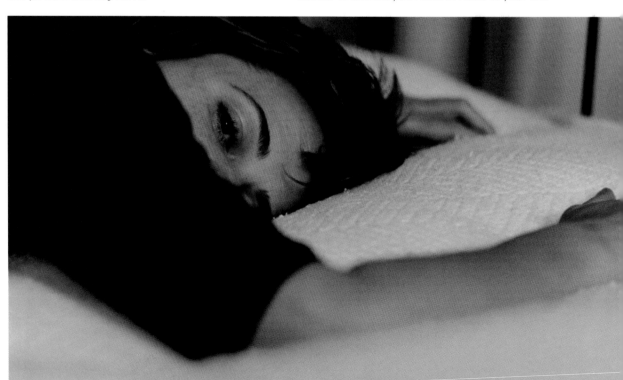

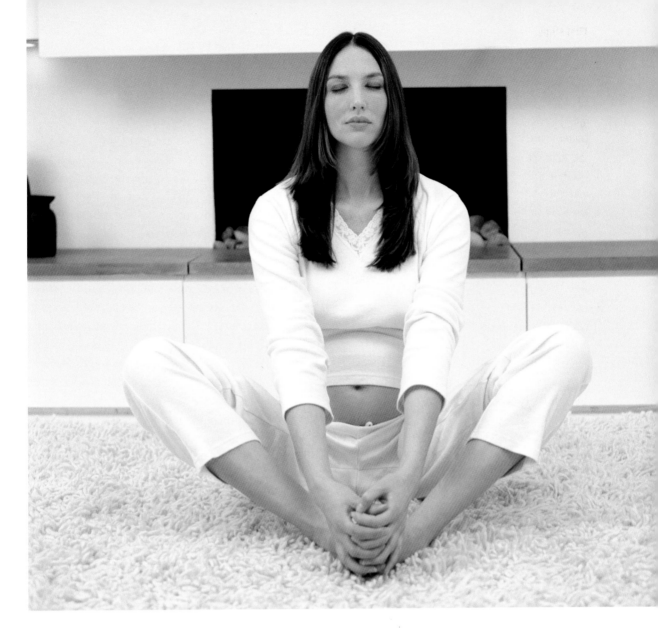

Fear of Change

Without your even realizing it, an unhealthy fear of change may be one of the most energy-depleting factors in your mental and emotional make-up. If you do suffer from a fear of change, it can apply to many aspects of your life. It can inhibit you from moving on and developing personal relationships, exploring important areas of your professional development or enjoying any of life's simple pleasures that flow from a healthy sense of spontaneity.

LEFT **FEELING LOW CAN MAKE YOU FEEL THAT YOU WANT TO RETREAT FROM OTHER PEOPLE.**
ABOVE **POSITIVE TIME SPENT RELAXING CAN RECHARGE YOUR MENTAL AND EMOTIONAL BATTERIES.**

If you feel that a basic anxiety has been instilled in you from childhood by parents who have unwittingly passed on their anxieties about change to you, you are likely to benefit from some professional help. This anxiety can manifest itself in anything from an obsessive fear of ageing to you becoming jittery or irritable if plans are changed at the last minute. General counselling may not be quite enough if your resistance to change is having a major, inhibiting effect on your life; you may find that you make more progress with a behavioural psychological approach such as cognitive therapy.

This can be an extremely liberating therapy, as it can enable you to identify patterns of behaviour that were laid down in your early, formative years. These

39

subconscious patterns can determine how we respond as adults to basic life challenges such as embracing change. Once you understand why these patterns are there, you are in the positive position of being able to break them if you choose to. As soon as this is within your grasp, it can free up an enormous amount of emotional and mental energy that you can use to enrich your life.

Inertia

It can be a persistent thread that runs throughout our lives, or inertia can be a feeling that emerges at certain key points in an otherwise stimulating life. These flash points are likely to occur at certain phases of life development or a major change in direction and/or pace. Times when a sense of general inertia can set in include becoming a parent for the first time (especially if this involves taking time out from a stimulating job), menopause, demotion, feeling caught on a stressful professional treadmill in order to keep up with financial commitments, 'downshifting', retirement or redundancy.

The risks involved in a sense of inertia carrying on for too long include lack of sparkle, a reduced sense of creativity, a general sense of fatigue and problems developing into actual depression. If a sense of inertia is more than a passing phase in your life – something that can hit any of us at any time in the natural course of events – you need to take action in order to reverse the negative trend.

If you want to break free from the paralysis of a creeping sense of inertia, you need to evaluate realistically the various possibilities at your disposal for injecting a sense of renewal and vitality into your professional and home lives. Depending on your individual situation, this could involve specific goal setting, asking for extra help so that you can delegate more effectively, instilling a sense of renewed physical energy through becoming physically fit, seeking professional advice to help you sort out financial problems, or asking for help in childminding from friends or family members so that you can have time for yourself outside home commitments.

Always keep in mind that your main objective in this exercise is to develop the capacity to think laterally. Consider all your options – you may be pleasantly surprised by how much scope you have in your life for positive change.

Pessimism

The perspective we bring to any situation can have an astonishing bearing on the eventual outcome. Consequently, those of us who naturally bring an upbeat, positive approach to problem-solving are almost certain to find that life goes pretty smoothly. It is not that problems dissolve as if by magic, it's just that positive approaches tend to generate positive results. If you give off a positive aura, you are likely to find that others pick up on this and tend to become more good-humoured and amenable in return.

Sadly, the reverse is also true. Having a downbeat, pessimistic approach to life's challenges tends to be a self-fulfilling prophecy. If you automatically expect a negative outcome, you can quite unconsciously pass this expectation on. It's also often true that if you inevitably expect the worst-case scenario every time you are presented with a challenging situation you will not be able to pick up on positive opportunities as they present themselves. As a result, unbridled pessimism tends to lead you towards a deepening negative spiral, with each disappointing experience locking you further into this negative way of thinking.

If you have exhibited a pessimistic streak since your childhood and suspect that this may be a pattern of thinking that was instilled in you from an early age, you may well need professional help in the form of counselling or cognitive therapy. A psychological technique of this kind can be just what you need to provide you with the necessary momentum to break those ingrained habits that no doubt feel as though they are second nature.

If, however, you are generally upbeat and positive most of the time, but have been hit hard by a disappointment in life that has made you feel uncharacteristically pessimistic and gloomy, you may be able to turn the situation around more quickly. This is simply because you will be working from a more positive baseline of emotional experience. In a situation like this, any of the following strategies are certainly worth a try.

- Talk over how you're feeling with someone you can trust. Ideally, whomever you choose needs to be someone you feel relaxed with, but also someone who tends to have a positive rather than downcast perspective on life. Otherwise there's a chance that you will end up feeling even worse than when you started.

- If there's a specific situation that you suspect you're feeling needlessly negative about, it can help to sit down and make a list of both positive and negative aspects of the issue concerning you. Try to clear your mind before beginning (some of the relaxation techniques outlined in later chapters of this book will help with this), so that you can take as objective a view as possible. If you apply

a balanced perspective to the problem, you may find that there are more positive features than you first thought possible. On the other hand, you may discover that your negative instinct was in fact the right one and you will then be able as a result to take whatever necessary action is needed to resolve the dilemma.

- If feeling blue has come on after an upsetting experience, it can make a huge difference if you see an alternative or complementary therapist. A properly qualified homeopath, herbalist or naturopath should be trained in listening skills, as well as being able to prescribe an appropriate herbal or homeopathic mood-balancing medicine to get you over the hump.

- For additional help with a temporary sense of gloom, see the ten steps to positive thinking in chapter 6 on page 107.

BELOW WE ALL NEED FUN TIME WHEN WE CAN LET OUR HAIR DOWN AND APPRECIATE THE LIGHTER SIDE OF LIFE.

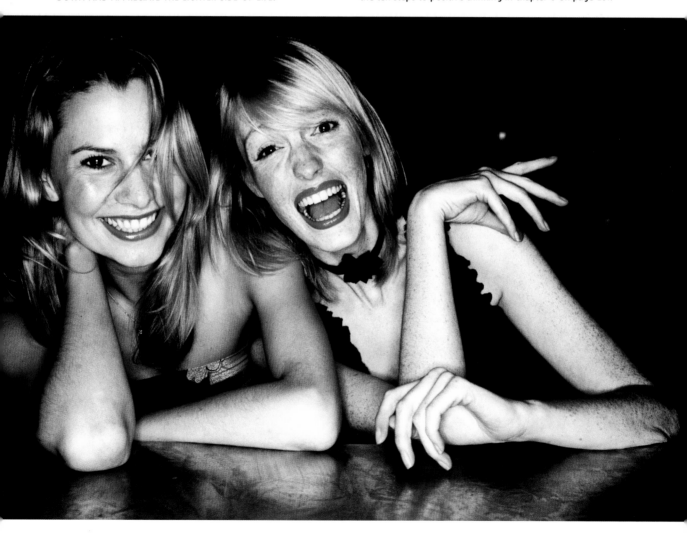

The Importance of Sound Sleep

Sound sleep is the foundation of smoothly flowing, well-balanced energy levels. Although we now understand a great deal about the mystery of sleep as a result of the information that has been generated from various sleep studies, the conclusions that have been drawn from this work can sometimes seem downright contradictory. A recent US study published in the *Archives of General Psychiatry* suggested, after examining the records of more than 1.1 million adults aged between 30 and 102, that the optimum amount of sleep associated with those who experienced a long life was six and a half hours a night. In other words, less sleep than was previously thought to be necessary for a healthy, relaxed night's rest. From this latest study, it has been concluded that the optimum amount of sleep a night to aim for should be around seven hours. Sleeping for a longer period of time each night appears to bring health disadvantages rather than health benefits.

On the other hand, a more recent report that appeared in the UK media drew attention to the serious problems that can be associated with experiencing not enough sleep. These include an increased risk of road-traffic accidents through drowsiness and reduced ability to respond quickly, as well as less dramatic but equally serious health-related problems. An increased predisposition to age-related conditions (high blood pressure and memory loss), mood swings, irritability, lack of concentration, indecisiveness and increased susceptibility to illness are just some of the downsides of not enough sleep.

If we take a balanced view of what we know about sleep so far, we appear to need the optimum amount of slumber that meets our individual needs. In other words, the number of hours' rest that helps us to wake refreshed and ready to face whatever each day holds in store for us. Within this context, talking about a specific, set goal can be meaningless, as some of us may instinctively know that we need eight hours of unbroken sleep in order to function at our

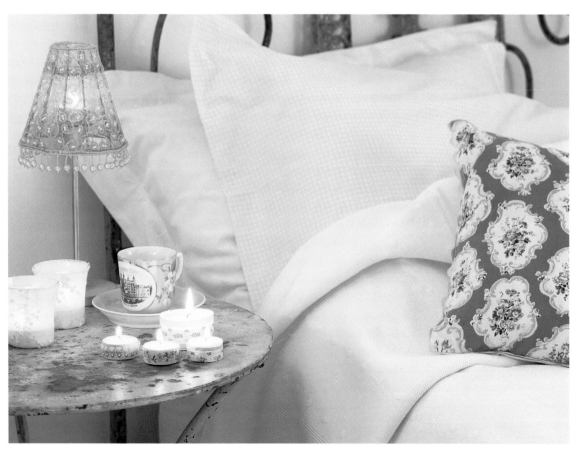

best, while others may be convinced that they feel great after just five hours. Any more and these people feel muzzy-headed and sluggish.

Whatever amount of sleep we require in order to meet our individual needs must be experienced regularly if we are to enjoy maximum health and vitality. As we have already seen, sleep deprivation can lead to a host of insidious health problems that can compromise everything from our mental and emotional balance to the effectiveness with which we fight off infection. In addition, enjoying regular, good-quality sleep is essential if we are to keep our energy levels topped up. This is partly related to the importance of giving our vital organs a chance to rest when we sleep, as they are known to work at a slower pace during this period.

If you are deprived of sleep for any extended length of time, you're also likely to find that you feel mentally tired and less capable of making clear, fast decisions. The sense of mental strain that can come about as a result of feeling mentally 'foggy' can be made even worse if you begin to react to lack of sleep by becoming irritable and short-tempered. By contrast, once you begin to enjoy regular sleep again, the benefits are enormous. Mental clarity, stable moods, a basic sense of relaxation and steady energy levels are all acknowledged benefits of a sound sleep pattern. Once your mental, emotional and physical energy levels have stabilized in response to a routine of regular, deep sleep, you should also find that you are less tempted to reach for chemical stimulants in the form of repeated cups of strong coffee to keep you functioning. This is obviously a significant health bonus in itself.

Relaxation, Nutrition, Regular Slumber and Alternative Remedies

By making an effort to put most of the following practical, sleep-promoting strategies in place, you should see an improvement in the overall quality and duration of your sleep in double-quick time.

LEFT **CREATING A SOOTHING, RELAXING ATMOSPHERE IN THE BEDROOM WILL HELP YOU TO DRIFT OFF TO SLEEP.**

Relaxation

One of the simplest yet most important ways of preparing for a sound night's refreshing sleep is to avoid doing anything that's demanding, stimulating or invigorating for at least a couple of hours before you go to bed. The biggest and often most tempting pitfall to avoid is working right up to the last minute before you attempt to fall asleep. The problems associated with this are pretty obvious really, as you need at least an hour of mental relaxation in order to prepare yourself to switch off mentally. Otherwise you are likely to find that your brain is still firing on all cylinders as your head hits the pillow.

Instead, make a point of doing something pleasurable and mentally relaxing for a couple of hours before retiring. This could involve reading a novel, listening to music, listening to a 'talking book', going through a guided relaxation exercise, taking a warm bath that has been scented with soothing aromatherapy oils or practising a relaxing breathing exercise. Activities to avoid near bedtime include taking any vigorous exercise, watching television (especially if the programme is nail-bitingly suspenseful) or having a heated argument, which is sure to raise adrenaline levels and make you feel wide awake, restless and anxious. Making love can either be sleep inducing or energizing, depending on your individual constitution. If you find that you feel deliciously relaxed and sleepy after making love, this can be one of the most pleasurable ways to drift off to sleep. On the other hand, if sex tends to make you feel euphoric and full of energy, it's probably best avoided last thing at night.

Nutrition

Those of us who are sensitive to stimulants such as caffeine or guarana should aim to avoid having any stimulating drinks from mid-afternoon onwards. Even if you boast the hardiest of constitutions you should avoid drinking coffee or strong tea after dinner: it may not obviously keep you awake, but it can still have an adverse effect on the depth of sleep that you enjoy.

Alcohol can also have a disturbing effect on your pattern of rest, making it less likely that you will reap the benefits of deep sleep. It helps to bear in mind that alcohol can be a mood enhancer, which is fine if you're feeling relaxed and positive before sleep, but becomes a problem when you're feeling anxious or jittery before going to bed. On a practical level, if you've had quite a few drinks of beer or wine before retiring, you're likely to find that you have to get up several times during the night to pass water. This will obviously hamper your attempt to achieve deep sleep.

You should also pay attention to the pattern of when you eat and drink, as well as the ingredients, for the timing and the amount of an evening meal can have a significant impact on the quality of sleep that you enjoy. One of the biggest mistakes that you can make is to eat a large, rich meal washed down with generous quantities of alcohol and coffee late at night. You will find sound sleep elusive owing to the sleep-disturbing effects of caffeine and alcohol. An additional problem is also likely to emerge, due to the way in which your digestive system functions at a slower rate when you sleep.

As a result of the resting mode that our major organs adopt when we sleep, basic body functions all operate at a slower rate. This need not cause any problems if your stomach is fairly empty and comfortable, but it can lead to great discomfort if you have a rich, three-course meal there needing to be broken down and digested. When this happens, you are likely to drop off to sleep fairly quickly, only to find to your dismay that you wake an hour or so later with a bout of severe indigestion, heartburn and/or queasiness. The best and most practical way of avoiding this is to eat in the early evening as a rule (it takes roughly up to four to six hours for food to be broken down in the stomach, depending on the contents). Alternatively, if you do eat later, make a point of avoiding red meat, cheese, cream and other full-fat ingredients that take longer to be broken down by stomach acids. Opt instead for items that are easy on your digestive system, including salads, grilled fish, chicken and boiled, steamed or stir-fried grains.

Surroundings

In order to sleep soundly and refreshingly, you need to feel both relaxed and secure. Following on from this, it makes a great deal of sense to pay attention to the atmosphere of your bedroom. Some of us may be experts at choosing an overall 'look' for our bedrooms that is visually very stunning, but forget to pay attention to the aspects of the room that will ensure we can actually relax there at night.

Although gauzy, light, filmy drapes and curtains look gorgeous, they won't do much to help you enjoy a sound night's sleep if you are woken easily by natural light streaming into the room. Extremely dark curtains should be avoided for the opposite reason, as they make it harder for you to wake refreshed and ready to face the day. Choose a colour, pattern and weight of fabric that filters enough bright light out to ensure that you don't wake too early.

It's also important to keep as much extraneous sound as possible out of the bedroom, especially if you are easily disturbed by the slightest noise. When moving to a new home, do consider carefully the position of the bedroom and how peaceful it is likely

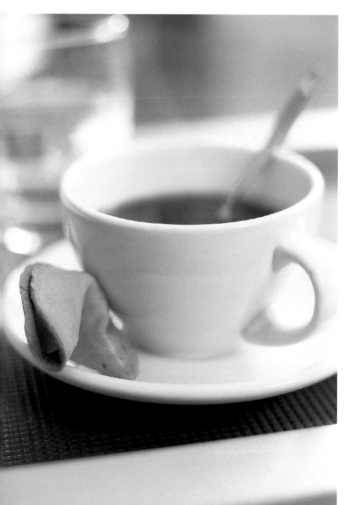

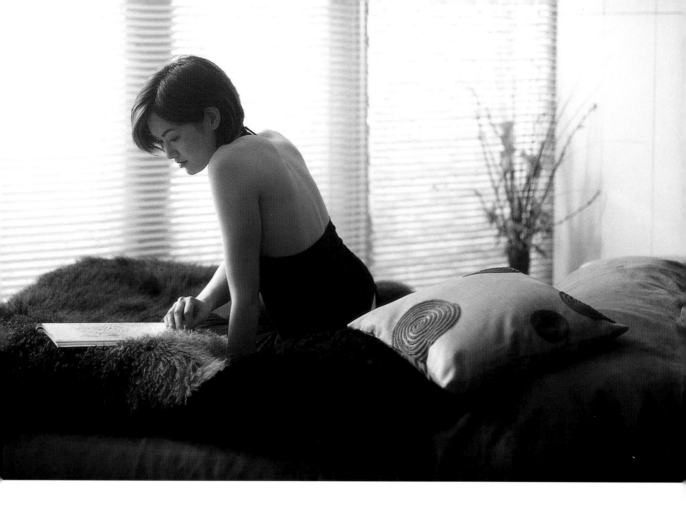

to be. If it overlooks a busy street, it may be worth relocating the bedroom to another room in a quieter position. If this just isn't practical, think about investing in double glazing to try to keep out as much sound as possible.

Routine

Take into account that sleep patterns tend to thrive on regular habit and that you really should give priority to establishing a regular sleep pattern. This is especially important at times of stress and pressure, or if you've been going through a phase of generally feeling rundown and mentally and physically tired. Of course, there will be times when life just doesn't

permit you to stick to a strict routine. And that's exactly as it should be, as a willingness to be flexible is a sign of a healthy lifestyle where there is always room for a burst of rejuvenating spontaneity. Yet this ready adaptability ideally needs to exist within a well-structured framework of a beneficial amount of routine. If your life becomes too irregular and chaotic, you're likely to put yourself at real risk of entering the sort of negative energy spiral outlined in the previous chapter (see pages 15–16).

Aim to establish a regular routine at bedtime so that your body recognizes that it's time to begin the process of mentally and physically winding down. Try to stick to a similar time for retiring at night that you instinctively feel is your optimum moment for drifting into a deep sleep. Over time, your body will become used to this rhythm of rest, and you should find it progressively easier to fall asleep and generally less difficult to wake up on time in the morning. Regular, unbroken, good-quality sleep of this kind pays huge dividends in the energy stakes, especially when you're under pressure.

LEFT **TEA AND COFFEE WILL DO NOTHING TO HELP YOU TO SWITCH OFF AND ENJOY A REFRESHING NIGHT'S REST. IF YOU DO WANT A HOT DRINK BEFORE BED, A SOOTHING HERBAL OR FRUIT TEA MAKES A GOOD CHOICE AS A NIGHTCAP.**
ABOVE **AVOID WORKING UNTIL THE VERY LAST MINUTE BEFORE FALLING INTO BED. IT IS A MUCH BETTER IDEA TO UNWIND FOR A COUPLE OF HOURS BEFORE RETIRING.**

Alternative and Complementary Remedies

If you have hit temporary problems with your sleep pattern or sleep quality, you will want to get things back on track as fast as possible. Alternatively, you may have had recurrent problems with a poor sleep history but definitely want to avoid dependence on conventional sleeping tablets. In both these cases you can benefit immensely from exploring the possibilities offered by alternative or complementary medicines. The help available from an alternative source is impressively free from risks of side effects and addiction, while providing gentle and effective results. If your sleep problems are well established and alternative medical help is being now sought in order to wean yourself off conventional sleeping tablets, it is strongly recommended to seek professional advice and support from a fully trained and qualified practitioner. Suitable therapies to investigate include homeopathy, naturopathy, Western medical herbalism, traditional Chinese medicine, ayurveda and hypnotherapy.

On the other hand, shorter-lived, less established sleep disturbance that can be traced to a specific recent period of stress or trauma may be helped considerably by the judicious use of alternative or complementary medicines at home. For a list of the possibilities, and instructions on how to select the most appropriate option and dosage, see the section on insomnia on page 114.

Don't Rely on the Adrenaline Rush

However exciting it may feel to spend time in the fast lane, the price you pay for living on high adrenaline surges to keep you moving and motivated is that you will inevitably stall at some point. When this eventually happens, you're likely to feel exhausted, irritable, moody and general off colour. Some of us may make the mistake of avoiding this 'crash and burn' scenario by relying on chemical stimulants to keep going and ensuring that levels of circulating adrenaline remain high through constantly putting ourselves under escalating pressure. This situation can have pretty disastrous consequences in the long run if it's allowed to continue for an extended period of time. You are eventually likely to display signs of adrenal exhaustion, no matter how many stimulants you pump into your system. When you're well on the way to this stage, common symptoms include poor concentration, mental and physical fatigue, muscle weakness, impaired resistance to infection, low blood pressure, palpitations and anxiety and/or depression.

As you can see, it makes a great deal of sense to pick up on any signals that suggest that you are heading for even an early stage of adrenal exhaustion so as to turn the situation around as quickly as you can. By making positive changes, you will be taking vital action that should bolster your energy reserves at a basic level, as well as reducing the likelihood of ending up with a chronic fatigue problem. Each of the following strategies should help.

Taking Control

Take a long, hard look at the balance between work and leisure hours in your life. If you discover that work has invaded more and more of your home life – whether because you have been taking large amounts of work home, working through weekends and/or staying at the office until late at night – it's time to take action. If delegating or saying no to extra tasks is a problem, take a look at the basic stress management advice given in the section below. Implementing the changes is bound to feel difficult or painful at first, but the physical and psychological health benefits that come from stepping off a relentless work treadmill are enormous. It also helps to know that taking the initial step is always the hardest part, as once the obvious benefits begin to emerge it becomes easier to stick to your resolve. Always remember that you don't have to go through this alone. Don't be afraid to ask for the support and backing of family members and friends, who will probably be delighted to help because it will mean that they will see more of you.

RIGHT **STEPPING OFF THE WORK TREADMILL AT FREQUENT AND REGULAR INTERVALS HELPS MAINTAIN HEALTHY BALANCE.**

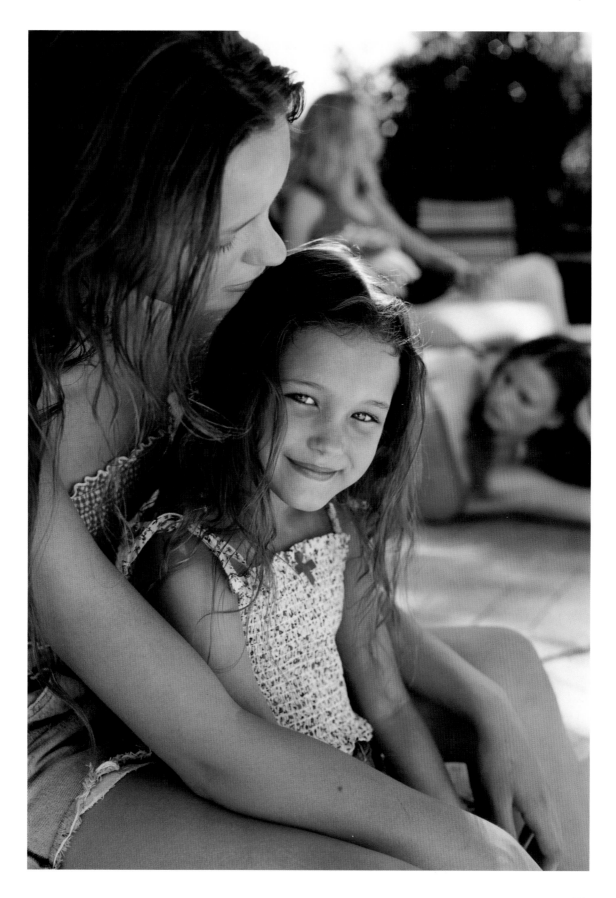

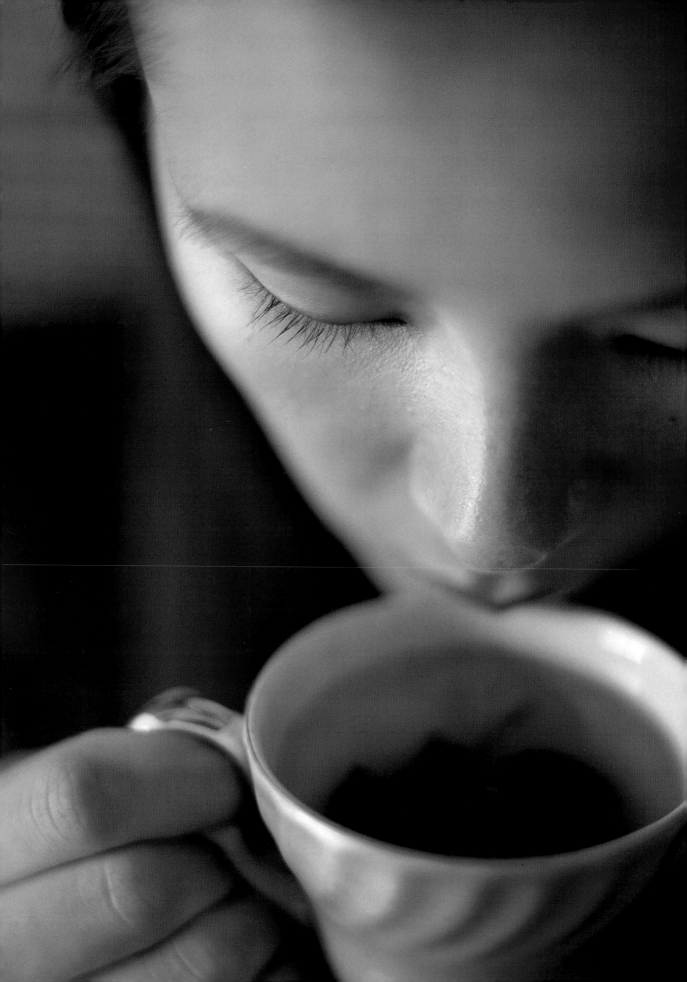

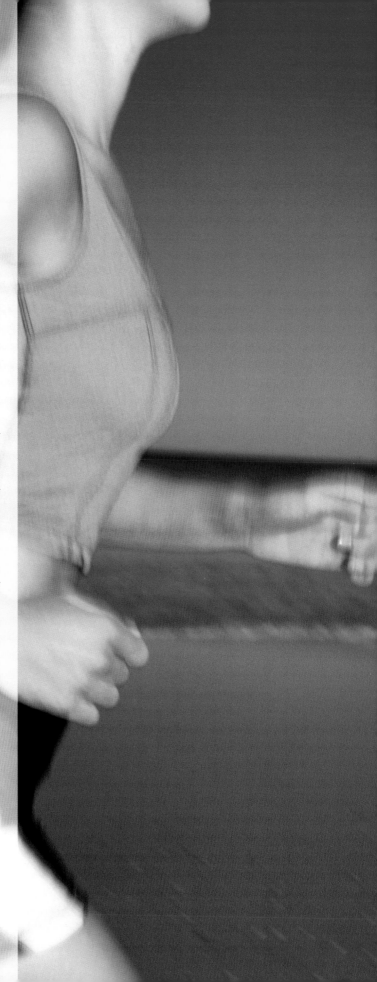

Kick the Stimulants

Reduce your intake of stimulants slowly and steadily in order to climb off that artificially induced energy rollercoaster. It is essential not to change too drastically or quickly, as caffeine withdrawal can feel really unpleasant, giving rise to symptoms including a severe headache, jitteriness and a generally 'toxic' feeling. Instead, aim to reduce your coffee, tea, and caffeinated soft drink intake gradually, introducing green, herbal or fruit teas, grain-based coffee substitutes, carbonated water or drinks flavoured with natural fruit and herbal extracts. Green teas can be especially helpful, as these provide a refreshing, invigorating alternative to black Indian or China tea that is both naturally low in caffeine and rich in antioxidants that will boost your immune system.

Get Moving

As you are likely to miss the lift and excitement of adrenaline surging through your system, it's very important to find alternative, health-promoting ways of giving yourself a feel-good boost. One of the most effective ways of achieving a natural high is taking regular, aerobic exercise, such as running, power walking, swimming, dancing or cycling. This natural emotional boost comes from the increased secretion and circulation of antidepressant chemicals in our bodies called endorphins. The secretion of these naturally occurring chemicals is known to be stimulated by vigorous, rhythmic exercise, so it makes sense to get moving if you've previously led a sedentary lifestyle and depended on adrenaline rushes and stimulants in order to feel alive.

Don't be put off by thinking that you have have to start by training for a half-marathon. You don't. Begin slowly with workable and achievable goals in mind. Above all, choose an activity you enjoy: you will be more likely to keep it up.

LEFT **GRADUALLY WEAN YOURSELF OFF CAFFEINATED DRINKS TO AVOID SYMPTOMS OF CAFFEINE WITHDRAWAL.** RIGHT **DON'T FORGET TO ENSURE THAT YOUR CHOICE OF EXERCISE IS FUN AS WELL AS GOOD FOR YOU.**

Learn to Switch Off

If you're used to living life in the fast lane, the last thing you're likely to be skilled at is the ability to switch off and replenish your energy reserves. This is an altogether different sensation from the absolute exhaustion you may be very familiar with when you have generally overdone things for too long. The art of relaxation is something that we all need to learn, and there is a host of ways of setting about doing so. This may include learning guided relaxation exercises, meditation, visualization techniques, yoga or perhaps t'ai chi. The choice is really down to you and your individual tastes, but you do need to find a method of effective relaxation that you can easily tap into on a daily basis. Once you have acquired the knack of becoming totally relaxed, you are likely to be amazed at the positive benefits you experience in the form of an enhanced ability to focus and concentrate, increased ability to sleep well, greater emotional stability and resilience, and freedom from general physical tension. All of these, in turn, have a positive effect on your baseline energy levels.

Tackling Poorly Managed Stress

These days, everyone seems to have opinions about stress. Some of us may think that it's one of the greatest blights on the horizon of 21st-century living, while others may vigorously defend the need for a high level of stress factors, as otherwise they fear being understimulated or bored.

As always, there is a very strong chance that the healthy answer to the stress problem lies somewhere in the middle. In other words, ensuring that you embrace enough positive stress in your professional and domestic lives to feel alive and motivated, but not so much that you feel swamped by impossible demands and run the risk of burn-out.

These concerns surrounding stress management have a particular relevance when it comes to any discussion about maintaining healthy, resilient energy levels. There is no doubt that excessive, unmanaged stress levels have a demonstrably draining effect on the amount of energy that you experience. This is partly due to the way in which worrying about issues

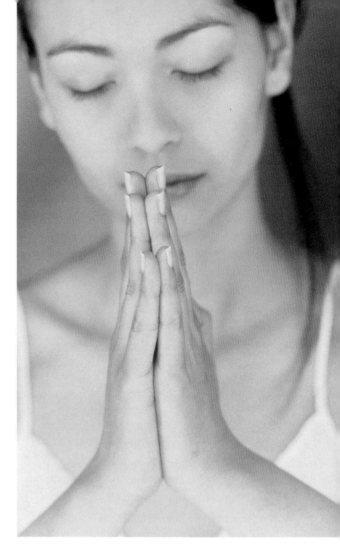

ABOVE **REGULAR PRACTICE OF MEDITATION IS ONE OF THE MOST EFFECTIVE STRESS-BUSTING TOOLS AT OUR DISPOSAL.**

in your life that are a focus of stress undoubtedly depletes your mental, emotional and physical vitality. This is even more the case if you feel helpless and powerless to take any positive steps to resolve the situation. When this happens, you go through the physiological effects of raised levels of adrenaline and cortisol, two of the best-known stress hormones, without having any outlet that will allow you to absorb or burn them off through positive action.

Yet once you take positive steps to deal with stress factors in your life, the practical benefits of feeling energized, more capable and confident, and experiencing an enhanced sense of relaxation once the issues have been dealt with are likely to follow rapidly. When these become a regular feature of your life, you are sure to find that your baseline levels of mental, emotional and physical energy improve. The natural consequence of this is that you should feel empowered to be more decisive and assertive.

It's therefore time to explore some basic stress-management techniques. Bear in mind that these are some of the most simple approaches of all. If you have success with these and feel the positive benefits that come from applying these basic principles, it would be well worth considering taking on board more sophisticated stress-management techniques such as those found in some of the titles listed at the back of this book (see page 124).

Never Put Off Till Tomorrow ...

This is probably the most essential basic stress-busting tactic we have at our disposal. Until you decide that action must be taken, you are never going to solve the problem. One of the most stressful things you can do is procrastinate and keep putting off tasks that must be tackled eventually. Unfortunately, while you're dodging confronting these jobs, your mind is still very aware of what you need to do and will be busily worrying about the situation, even if you're not always consciously aware of it. This scenario has a profoundly energy-draining effect, as you will usually find that you can't concentrate fully on whatever task you have in hand. It is also unlikely that you will be able to switch off completely at night. This will be especially true if you have a growing pile of jobs that need to be addressed – in time, this is going to prove an increasing psychological burden.

The good news, however, is that, once you take the vital first (though initially difficult) step, you will almost certainly discover a delightful secret: tackling whatever job you were putting off is never as difficult as you thought. This is mainly because anticipating a problem tends to exaggerate its proportions. Most of us find that once we've set the ball rolling, the task can be carried out much faster than we would have predicted – more often than not without most of the complications we envisaged. Even if problems do present themselves, though, solutions also have a happy habit of emerging that we were unable to imagine in our negative scenario because our minds were too preoccupied.

Prioritize

Those of us who are best at making friends with stress usually have an instinctive ability to cut through a maze of pressing tasks and be able to instinctively identify what needs to be tackled first. Don't worry if this hasn't been a frequent experience for you until now, as it is as much a skill that can be learnt and mastered as it is a natural attribute. If you are a newcomer to the skill of effective prioritizing, you need to explore the advantages of real listmaking. You are unlikely to have got very far if you've always previously relied on making mental lists. Mental lists lack clarity and focus – two essential stress-diffusing qualities – as they can constantly shift and change, according to how much emphasis you're putting on any item on that list at any given moment.

BELOW **MESSY SURROUNDINGS CAN AGGRAVATE A GENERAL SENSE OF FEELING STRESSED AND UNABLE TO COPE.**

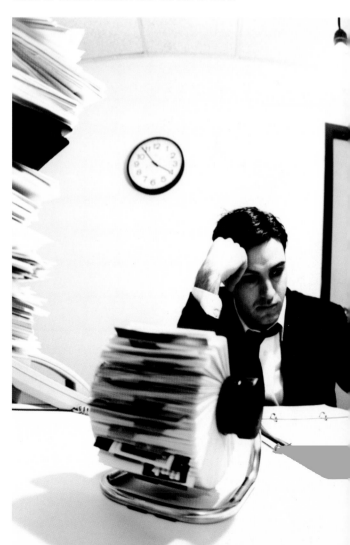

Producing a physical list, however, makes the issues that demand to be addressed much clearer. It can be very helpful to adopt an underlining system, giving those issues that demand urgent attention three lines, those that are important and pressing two lines, and those that can be tackled later one line. Make a point of ticking off items as they're dealt with, as this rewards you with a therapeutic glow from seeing tasks that may have been haunting you for ages finally dispensed with.

Delegate

Once you've learnt how to prioritize the tasks you're faced with, this must be backed up with effective delegating skills if you are to reap the maximum benefit of effective stress-management strategies. There's a very good chance that, apart from the important urgent jobs that must be carried out by you personally, there will also be less pressing jobs that could be appropriately passed on to others. Bear in mind that those of us who feel we must hang on to all the tasks that we are faced with, regardless of the fact that they could be done as effectively and much faster by others, often become the most stressed-out, exhausted people of all.

The first step to effective delegating is simply to let go and accept that it's not necessary to feel in control of every task, no matter how small and insignificant. Here again, those of us who find it very hard to ask for help often don't feel as calm and in as healthy and balanced a state of control as those who will readily part with extra tasks that don't require their personal attention and action.

The positive gains that come with learning and practising delegating skills are both immediate and obvious. Once you see that other people are often delighted to be asked to help (this applies as much at home and in the extended family as it does in the work context), you may begin to realize that you can safely share your responsibilities with those whom you trust. This, in turn, will eventually lead you to the liberating insight that you are not indispensable. As

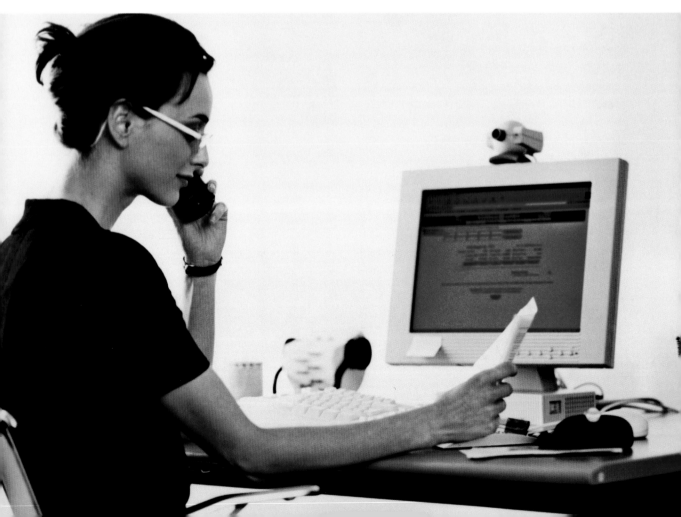

threatening as this realization may sometimes seem at first, in the long run most stressed-out individuals are relieved to discover that they don't actually have to carry the world on their shoulders.

Learn to Say No

Learning to say no isn't about avoiding issues and tasks that you need to confront and to deal with decisively – that would be a clear instance of the procrastination discussed earlier. Rather, this is about setting realistic, working boundaries so that you can be as creative and productive as possible, without taking on the burden of additional tasks that you know you don't have the time or expertise to accomplish. In many ways, what I am talking about here is an organic development borne from prioritizing skills. If you know that you're working productively to your healthy maximum, you need to be very firm about taking on any extra inappropriate work, however much subtle pressure may be applied. Remaining vigilant in this manner does an enormous amount to protect you from becoming burnt out. When you're tempted to do too much, think seriously about how much quality time you have for yourself. If this looks in danger of being squeezed in any way for too long, it's high time that you said no firmly and politely.

Organize

When that old, sinking feeling that you're finding it hard to cope sneaks up on you, stop whatever you're doing for a moment or two. Take a long, hard look around you. Often your external environment can very accurately reflect your state of mind. For instance, if you're suffering from a protracted, severe bout of depression, you may have begun to neglect your appearance and household chores, and simply want to retreat to bed. You may be reinforcing feelings of being stressed and unable to cope with

LEFT **THE IDEA OF CLEARING CLUTTER IS USUALLY MUCH MORE OFFPUTTING THAN THE REALITY OF DOING IT. ONCE YOU START ORGANIZING YOUR SURROUNDINGS, YOU WILL FEEL SO MUCH BETTER FOR IT THAT YOU WILL WANT TO CONTINUE THE EFFORT TO MAINTAIN THE IMPROVEMENT.**

surroundings that are disorganized, thereby making it even harder for you to get on with your task.

If you are surrounded by teetering stacks of papers piled high on your desk or a huge number of e-mails you haven't dealt with on your computer screen, this will probably reinforce all those lurking feelings of being disorganized and overwhelmed by the scale of what you have to deal with. Fortunately, once you begin to tackle your professional and domestic surroundings, you are likely to discover that functioning more efficiently and enthusiastically is not so impossible after all.

In a purely practical terms, you're going to find it so much easier and less maddening to knuckle down to creatively flowing work when you can locate the material that you need quickly and with only the minimum amount of fuss. Just take a moment to consider the flipside. You're going to waste a great deal of energy and time if you have to search through endless piles of paper until you eventually find what you're looking for. The very fact of quickly being able to lay your hands on something that you need without any fuss or hair tearing can shortcircuit those feelings of irritation and frustration that inevitably arise if you have lost a vital document when under the pressure of a tight deadline.

Always remember that what you're aiming for here is a healthy, balanced approach to clearing clutter, as an excessive preoccupation with neatness and organizing can become a mental and emotional straitjacket. If such a preoccupation remains unaddressed, then becoming obsessively focused on tidiness can become a sad reality. Once things have reached this point, the sheer compulsion to maintain order and control can lead you to spend more time and effort on preparing tasks than on completing them – an act of self-sabotage if ever there were one.

Once you reach a healthy point of balance with regard to organizing yourself, you can consolidate your achievement by resolving in future always to take action to diffuse stress levels and to prevent you from putting things off indefinitely. Being proactive in this way gives your self-esteem a huge boost, which in turn can have a very positive effect on mental and emotional energy.

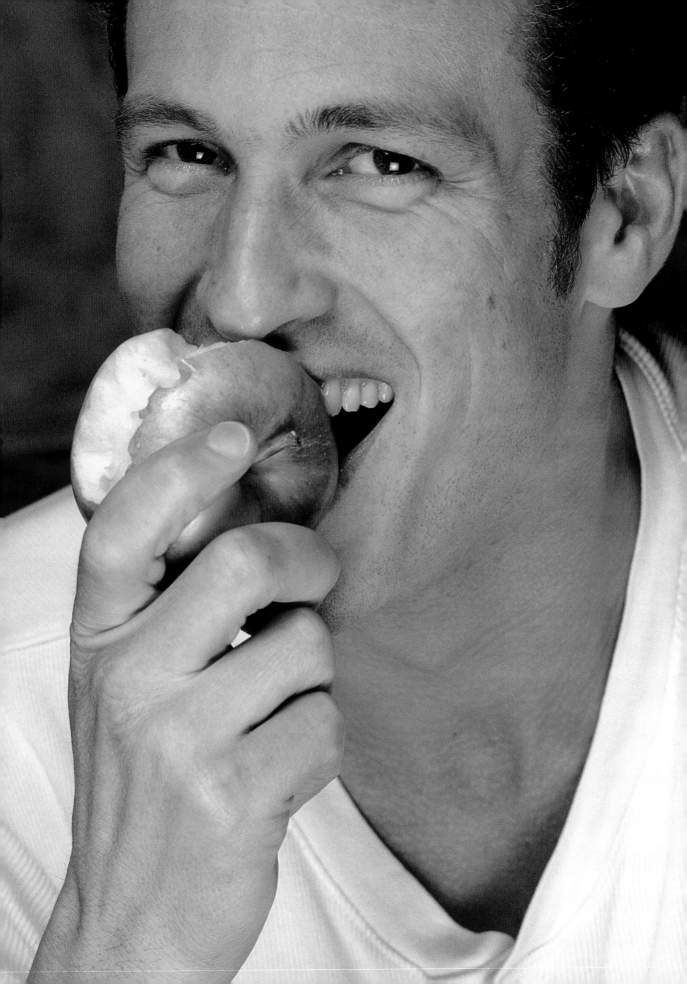

3 Nurturing energy

As clichéd as it undoubtedly sounds, we really are what we eat. The quality and quantity of food and liquid that we enjoy on a regular basis has a huge impact on our psychological health. What we ingest also affects the amount of energy we have, our ratio of body fat to lean muscle, and the general level of health that we enjoy from day to day.

Of course, eating is about so much more than providing basic building blocks and fuel for our bodies. If this were all we had to worry about, we might as well all just take carefully nutritionally engineered supplements to meet our daily requirements. Apart from becoming incredibly boring, this approach would deny the fact that eating is one of the most enjoyable experiences for our senses that is available to us. The smell, texture, appearance and taste of food can be incredibly pleasure-giving, becoming even more so when we enjoy meals in the company of those we love.

Sadly, there are other aspects of eating that can be less than life-enhancing, as many of us may find ourselves caught up in guilt trips over eating too much, too often, too little, or just too unhealthily. These issues can often come to the fore when other aspects of life aren't going well, so you may find yourself reaching for chocolate bars or jumbo packets of corn chips not because you feel the rumbles of real hunger pangs, but because you're in search of comfort. Of course, once you've finished eating you embark on another guilt trip, and so the cycle continues. Once you gain an understanding of how the quality and amount of food that you eat can have a profound effect on your mental, emotional and physical health and basic sense of wellbeing, however, you are in a powerful position to take action to improve your situation.

This should be a particular priority for anybody who suffers from low or erratic energy levels, as the food and drinks you consume on a daily basis can have a huge impact on the amount of energy at your disposal. In many ways, establishing healthy eating patterns is one of the most pivotal steps that you can take on the path to high-energy living.

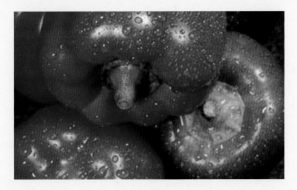

LEFT **EAT AT LEAST FIVE PORTIONS OF FRESH FRUIT AND VEGETABLES A DAY FOR MAXIMUM HEALTH AND VITALITY.** RIGHT **BRIGHT RED, ORANGE, YELLOW AND DARK GREEN VEGETABLES ARE AN IMPORTANT SOURCE OF ANTIOXIDANTS.**

NUTRITION AND ENERGY PRODUCTION

When thinking about the relationship between what you regularly eat and the amount of baseline vitality that you experience, visualize your body as a high-performance car and the foods and drinks that make up your daily diet as fuel. In other words, would you expect to get the best out of a Porsche if it were driven on the lowest-grade fuel? The same principle applies to your body, as the food that you eat every day has to be broken down to provide the building blocks that will repair old cells and make new ones, while at the same time providing energy and heat.

In other words, what you eat and drink regularly will determine how well your body performs at the most basic of levels. So it makes sense to ensure that you are getting the full complement of nutrients on a daily basis that you need to sustain optimum health and energy. The list of requirements includes vitamins, enzymes, minerals, amino acids, essential fatty acids, antioxidants, fibre and plenty of water.

You also need to take into account that at certain times of life your nutritional needs will change owing to extra demands being made on your body (e.g. during pregnancy, puberty or menopause, following a drastic weight-loss plan or when you experience great stress). Bearing this in mind, it makes sense to protect your baseline nutritional status on a long-term basis, so that when you hit extra-demanding phases you are able to roll with the punches without feeling exhausted and wrung out.

Bringing your nutritional status as much into line as possible should deliver a huge additional bonus. Any minor health problems that may have been compromising your baseline energy levels and generally making you feel under par should clear up. Recurrent headaches, indigestion, constipation, poor skin tone, mood swings and a disturbed sleep pattern can all benefit from improving the pattern and overall quality of what you eat and drink regularly.

As we shall see in the sections below, this chapter is all about getting the core principles right, so that you can adopt this style of eating as your basic framework from now on. Care has been taken when formulating the guidance to make it as flexible and enjoyable as possible, so that making a commitment to stick to it will not be so onerous. As a result, much of the advice relates to items that you can add to your diet rather than listing prohibited foods. In the small number of cases where specific foods or drinks need to be eliminated, plenty of healthy replacements are always mentioned. After all, eating should be an enjoyable experience rather than a guilt-inducing or punishing one. Attention is also drawn to the significance of eating patterns (the frequency or regularity with which you eat or drink). This is an extremely important factor to consider when aiming to sustain high-quality energy levels. It is particularly so at times of high stress, when there is a strong temptation to skip meals or grab a quick-fix snack. If this happens infrequently, it shouldn't cause major problems, but once it becomes an established pattern, digestive troubles are sure to follow.

Although these general nutritional boundaries will be broadly suitable for anyone, specific dietary advice applying to the constitutional types outlined in chapter 1 (pages 24–31) is also given.

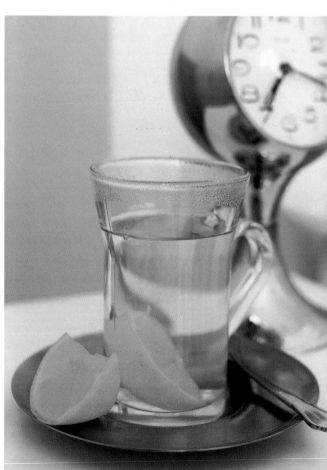

AVOIDING THE ENERGY ROLLER COASTER

Zappers

There is an awful lot of confusion surrounding the dietary items discussed in this section, as they are often thought of as the automatic things to reach for when you need a quick-fix energy boost. While it's true that in the short term these foods and drinks can give you a shot of increased energy, you pay a high price in the health stakes if you rely on them in large quantities for too long. They are really counterproductive in the long run, having a negative effect on your overall energy levels and contributing to making you feel moody, unable to concentrate, jittery and prone to rapidly developing episodes of exhaustion. You can get away with resorting to some of them in small quantities on an occasional basis, but the following should be treated with caution if you're concerned about boosting your basic sense of vitality in the long term. When cutting down or eliminating these items from your diet, substitute healthier ones so that you don't end up feeling deprived.

Sugar

Many of us still mistakenly think that whenever we feel we can't keep up the pace, the best way of giving ourselves a quick-fix energy boost is to increase our sugar intake. While a sugar 'rush' undoubtedly does give us the temporary lift we are after, the problem is that the effect is short lived. What is worse is that a high sugar intake results in ever-repeating peaks and troughs of energy. It also leads to a host of health problems including weight gain, increased risk of developing type II diabetes, dental cavities, thrush (*Candida albicans*), increased mucus production and a depressed immune system function, which in turn renders the body prone to recurrent infections.

LEFT **TRY BLENDS OF FRUIT-FLAVOURED TEAS IF YOU PREFER A SHARPER TASTE TO SOME OF THE SUBTLE HERBAL FLAVOURS.** RIGHT **SWEETS AND CANDIES DO NOTHING FOR OUR HEALTH IN GENERAL AND PLAY A MAJOR ROLE IN TOOTH DECAY.**

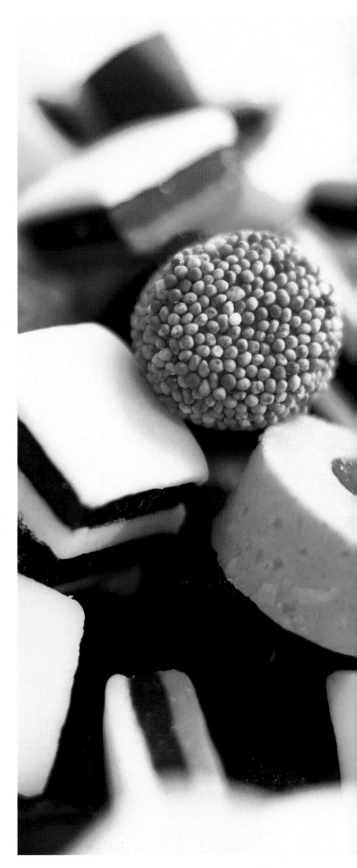

It helps to remember that refined white sugar (the sort that is used in large quantities in biscuits and cookies, cakes, chocolate bars and carbonated drinks) is a nutritionally 'empty' ingredient. In other words, the nutrients you use up to break down foods that are high in refined sugar are not replaced by the sugar itself. As a result, you're left with a nutritional deficit, rather than a gain.

In addition, there are more serious problems associated with regular, high consumption of refined sugar. These are linked to the way our bodies react to an influx of sweetened foods and drinks. At first you feel energized by a sharp rise in blood sugar, but your body quickly responds to this rapid rise in blood sugar levels by wanting to bring them back down again. This is achieved through the secretion of insulin by the pancreas, which lowers blood sugar levels promptly. This should not be too much of a problem if it is an infrequent occurrence, but, if it happens on a regular basis, it puts your pancreas under a huge

strain. Once you reach a point where the pancreas simply cannot cope any more (insulin resistance), you are at great risk of diabetes setting in.

If you don't understand what's happening when your blood sugar levels drop in response to the secretion of insulin, you're likely mistakenly to interpret this sense of a slowing down of pace as a signal that you need more sugar to give you another lift. If you do this, the same process repeats itself, until you're eventually going to find yourself on a very uncomfortable energy rollercoaster. Sadly, you're also going to discover that you need ever larger doses of refined sugar to achieve the same 'rush', so your tastebuds will crave increasingly sweet flavours.

If you want to reduce your overall intake of refined white sugar, bear in mind that, apart from the obvious sources such as granulated sugar, cakes, desserts, sweets (candies) and syrups, there are all sorts of foods and drinks that contain 'hidden' sugars. These traps include the following: breakfast cereals,

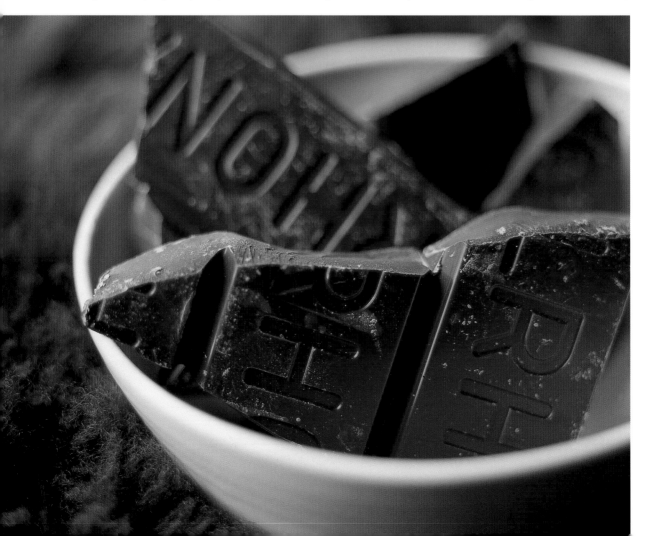

baked beans, tomato ketchup, convenience foods, mayonnaise, chutneys and pickles. While not all forms of sugar have such a destabilizing effect on your energy levels, if you want to get to grips with chronically low energy levels, you do need to jettison as many sources of refined white sugar as possible.

Caffeinated Drinks

Here we are essentially looking at coffee, tea and carbonated cola drinks. Although these are often the most common drinks we reach for when we're feeling tired and sluggish in the middle of the day and want a quick boost of energy, relying on this strategy to get by brings a multitude of problems with it. These include a tendency to feel jittery, on edge, short-tempered and generally extremely irritable. Too much caffeine circulating throughout your system on a regular basis also leads to sleep problems, chronic indigestion, palpitations (awareness of an irregular, rapid heartbeat) and heightened anxiety.

As if this weren't enough to deal with, caffeine has an adverse effect on blood sugar levels as well. A cup or two of espresso will raise those levels, an effect that is exacerbated if you also eat a few biscuits (cookies) or a chocolate bar with that cup of coffee or strong tea. If you have a combined high intake of caffeinated drinks and sugar, you're almost certainly going to experience the irregular energy pattern outlined above. Regular consumption of caffeinated drinks kicks our adrenal glands into action as well. Once you move into a state of adrenal exhaustion, you will be prone to bouts of extreme mental, emotional and physical fatigue. As our adrenal glands are involved in the secretion of stress hormones, however tempting it is to give yourself a shot of caffeine when you're under pressure, do your utmost to resist, as this will only make the situation worse in the long run.

Fizzy colas with added caffeine also bring their own special problems, which make them an unwise choice when you're trying to improve your health

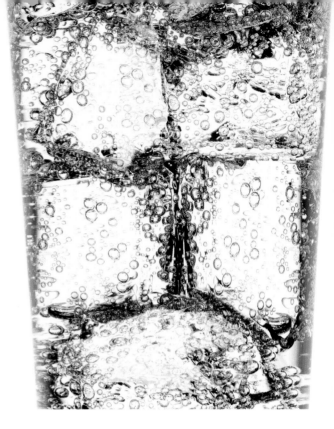

and boost or balance your energy levels. These carbonated drinks have very little going for them apart from the flavour, as they tend to be a cocktail of sugar, artificial sweeteners, flavourings and colourings, with a dash of caffeine added for good measure. Apart from raising blood sugar levels abruptly (owing to the combination of sugar and caffeine), these drinks can lead to problems with weight gain, elevated risk of osteoporosis because of the phosphorus content of many carbonated soft drinks, and increased likelihood of dental cavities.

Something else to bear in mind is that caffeinated drinks are diuretic in action (in other words, they encourage the body to eliminate fluid). If you're unaware of this, you may mistakenly think that you're having a decent intake of fluid each day because you have seven or eight teas or coffees a day. however, if you aren't taking generous amounts of water each day on top of this, you're likely to be in a low-grade state of dehydration without even realizing it. If this has become an ongoing problem, you're likely to experience the tell-tale symptoms of recurrent headaches, constipation, dry, poor skin tone and low energy levels. Such low-level dehydration can also aggravate an underlying tendency to retain fluid, as the body tries to conserves its reserves of water.

LEFT **CHOCOLATE SHOULD BE AN INFREQUENT INDULGENCE RATHER THAN A DAILY PART OF YOUR DIET.**

ABOVE RIGHT **SUGARY FIZZY DRINKS ARE BEST AVOIDED.**

Alcohol

In moderation, the occasional glass of red wine can be a pleasant, health-supporting experience. Some have suggested that, because it is the antioxidant reservatrol found on the skin of grapes that appears to be responsible for the beneficial effects on our circulatory system, we would be better off just eating the grapes and thus avoiding the negative effects of the alcohol. While this is, strictly speaking, quite true, it doesn't take into account the fact that an occasional glass of good-quality wine savoured over a delicious meal with friends can be an immensely convivial, pleasurable experience. Sadly, tucking into a bunch of grapes somehow doesn't give quite the same glow.

Having said this, if your consumption of alcohol should ever go beyond the infrequent stage, you're likely to pay a heavy price with regard to your energy levels. An overgenerous intake of alcohol is known to have an adverse effect on your sleep quality and pattern, psychological balance, concentration and digestion. This is partly due to the strain that regular alcohol consumption puts on the liver, and partly linked to the well-known way in which alcohol raises blood sugar levels in much the same fashion as sugar and caffeine. As a result, when you come down, you're likely to feel more exhausted than you did before you felt the temporary lift. On top of all this, regular high consumption of alcohol can deplete the body of a range of vitamins, including vitamin C, an effect that is much more marked if you smoke as well as drink regularly. It's also crucial to remember that alcohol is a powerful mood intensifier. As a result, you should always avoid it if you're feeling emotionally low. After the initial feeling of relaxation that comes with a drink of alcohol, you will soon begin to feel even more blue than you did in the first place.

If you want to enjoy optimum mental, emotional and physical energy, it makes a great deal of sense to treat alcohol with respect. It's also a good idea to avoid drinking even a small amount of alcohol every single day, as your liver will benefit greatly from being given an occasional rest. Thankfully there are healthy choices we can make in preference to automatically downing a few glasses of alcohol with a meal.

Refined Carbohydrates

Any of the following are refined carbohydrates: white bread, white rice, white pasta, white sugar and any other products made from white flour such as cakes and snack foods. These items have generally been bleached and milled to the point where they have lost most of their natural fibre, vitamin and mineral content, so they are broken down rapidly by your body. Consequently, they can raise your blood sugar levels swiftly, leading to peaks and troughs of energy. As we shall see below, the trick to sustaining energy levels doesn't involve avoiding carbohydrates completely. It's more a question of choosing the right kind of carbohydrate.

Cigarettes

Although not a food item, it is worth pausing for a brief moment to consider why cigarettes can have an energy-depleting effect on your body. We must all know by now the general health problems are that are associated with smoking (increased risk of heart disease, cancer, hardening of the arteries, high blood pressure, osteoporosis and lung diseases such as emphysema). However, smoking also has a powerful effect on free radical production in your body. Free radicals are naturally occurring, rampaging molecules that have a hugely destructive effect on overall health. The results can include any of the following: visible signs of early ageing, increased risk of heart disease, poor circulation, reduced mental performance and generally poor immune system functioning. None of these is going to do anything to enhance your basic sense of vitality, so you would do your body a huge favour all round if you kick the cigarette habit.

Boosters

These are the foods and drinks that must form the framework of your eating habits. All of the boosters mentioned on the following pages play an important part in providing you with the nutritional building blocks your body needs in order to enjoy balanced, sustained, high energy levels. The body's need for the support that these items supply will increase at times of stress and mental and physical pressure.

Water

It has been estimated that our bodies are made up of roughly 70 per cent fluid. As a result, while you can do without food for a reasonably lengthy period of time, once you become severely dehydrated you will die astonishingly quickly. Fortunately, unless we become seriously ill or suffer from severe heat stroke, most of us aren't at risk of severe dehydration in our daily lives. But without being conscious of it, you may be compromising your baseline levels of vitality by lurching through each day at a low-grade level of dehydration. This imposes a continual strain on your eliminatory organs (including the kidneys and bowel) that can make you feel tired, muzzy-headed and headachey on a frequent basis. The problem may be exacerbated even more if you frequently rely on the diuretic drinks discussed earlier to give you a temporary energy boost.

Once you take action by drinking at least five large glasses of filtered tap water or still mineral water a day, you will experience benefits that may surprise you. Bowel function should improve enormously, making you feel less sluggish immediately as a result, while your skin tone should become fresher and clearer. Nagging problems that may have been present (such as a tendency to intermittent bouts of cystitis) may also disappear as if by magic, while daily headaches that may have developed habitually as the day progressed may also clear up. All as a payoff for drinking more water.

Don't fall into the common trap of thinking that you can rely on your thirst mechanism to tell you when you need water. Some of us are thirsty by nature, but you may be one of the many people who don't feel any marked need for a drink until they have reached a pronounced stage of dehydration. Always make a point of drinking a large glass of water when you wake up, followed by another mid-morning, mid-afternoon, late afternoon and early evening. Although it's usually best to stick to still water, you can introduce variety by adding a twist of lemon or lime, or have the occasional drink of sparkling mineral

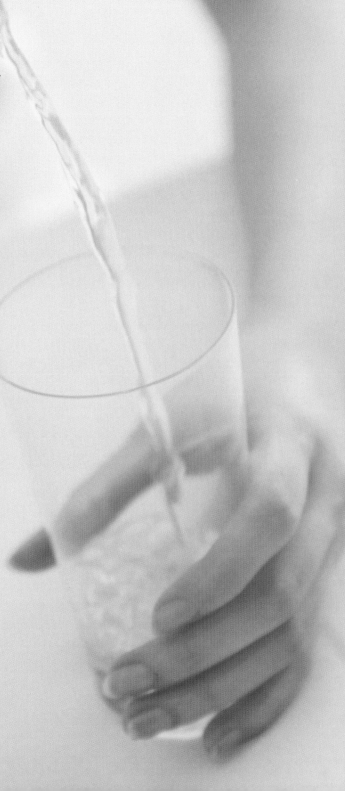

RIGHT **KEEP A BOTTLE OF WATER NEAR BY, AND MAKE A HABIT OF DRINKING AT REGULAR INTERVALS DURING THE DAY.**

water. If you're prone to feeling gassy or bloated, it's wise not to overdo the carbonated water.

A helpful habit to acquire is to drink a large glass of water after every cup of tea, coffee or chocolate, or a glass of alcohol. This is a simple, practical way of replacing the fluid that these drinks will encourage your body to eliminate.

Unrefined Carbohydrates

Some of the best, slow-release, energy-sustaining foods that you can eat are unrefined carbohydrates. This is mainly thanks to their fibre content, which acts as an important buffer to their being broken down in the digestive tract; however, it is also due to the fact that they are nutritionally intact. This is because they haven't been milled, bleached and generally chemically refined out of existence – unlike the items made from refined carbohydrates listed on page 60.

As a result, unrefined carbohydrates are often described as 'whole' foods because they are as packed with nutritional value as the basic amount of processing they are subjected to will allow them to be. The items that will keep your energy levels as stable as possible while providing you with a wide range of vitamins and minerals, fibre and slow-release sugars include the following superstars: wholemeal (wholewheat) bread, wholemeal (wholewheat) pasta, brown rice, chickpeas, lentils, beans and starchy vegetables such as potatoes eaten with the skin intact. The energy-balancing effect of these foods is likely to be enhanced when they're combined with small portions of protein such as fish, eggs, poultry, pulses and modest servings of favourite cheeses (preferably low in fat).

BELOW **WHOLEMEAL OR WHOLEGRAIN BREAD IS A DELICIOUS SOURCE OF SLOW-RELEASE CARBOHYDRATE, WHICH HELPS TO KEEP YOUR BLOOD SUGAR LEVELS STABLE.**

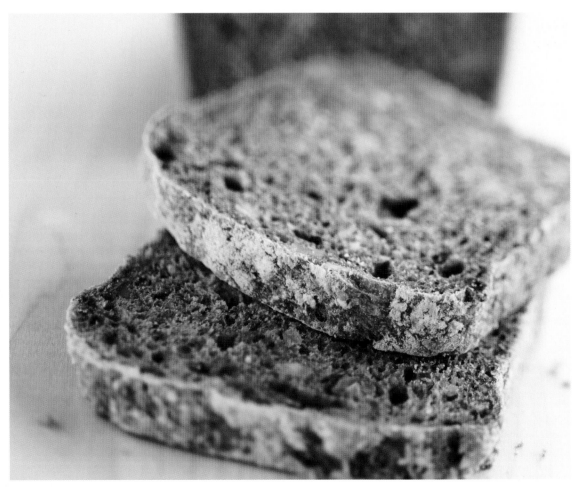

Raw Foods

Raw, fresh vegetables and fruit have a major role to play in stimulating high-level health and vitality. In particular, dark green, orange, red and yellow fruit and vegetables are packed with antioxidant nutrients that help to minimize the havoc that can be wreaked on your body by free radical activity. Vitamin C is one of the best-known antioxidants and acts as a sort of 'search and destroy' agent when any free radicals come into contact with it.

Antioxidants constitute invaluable allies, boosting your immunity to infection, protecting your heart and circulatory system, and also reducing the risk of degenerative problems developing such as memory loss and signs of premature ageing. Although we can supplement these nutrients in tablet or capsule form, this is really no substitute for getting them through increasing our intake of fresh, raw foods. Raw ingredients that are rich in antioxidants also have high-fibre contents (which guards against the fruit sugar of naturally sweet fruit entering your bloodstream too quickly, as refined sugar does). Eating a piece of fruit will give you a healthy energy boost when you feel that you're flagging, with a significantly reduced risk of roller-coasting peaks and troughs following as a result.

If you increase your intake of fresh vegetables and fruit on a regular basis, you should also find that you experience other health bonuses, such as enhanced resistance to infections such as colds, coughs and stomach bugs, and fewer problems with constipation. These bonuses are also likely to make you feel generally much perkier and full of vitality.

If you want to maximize the benefits that come from a high antioxidant yield in your diet, make a point of including regular helpings of the following fruits and vegetables in your meals every day, and be sure to vary them: raw green peppers, parsley, watercress, strawberries, watermelon, peaches, blackcurrants, broccoli, cauliflower, sprouts, nuts (unroasted and unsalted), lemons, oranges, whole grains, carrots, sweet potatoes, spinach, tomatoes, asparagus and apricots.

RIGHT **ARTICHOKES ARE A GOOD SOURCE OF POTASSIUM.**

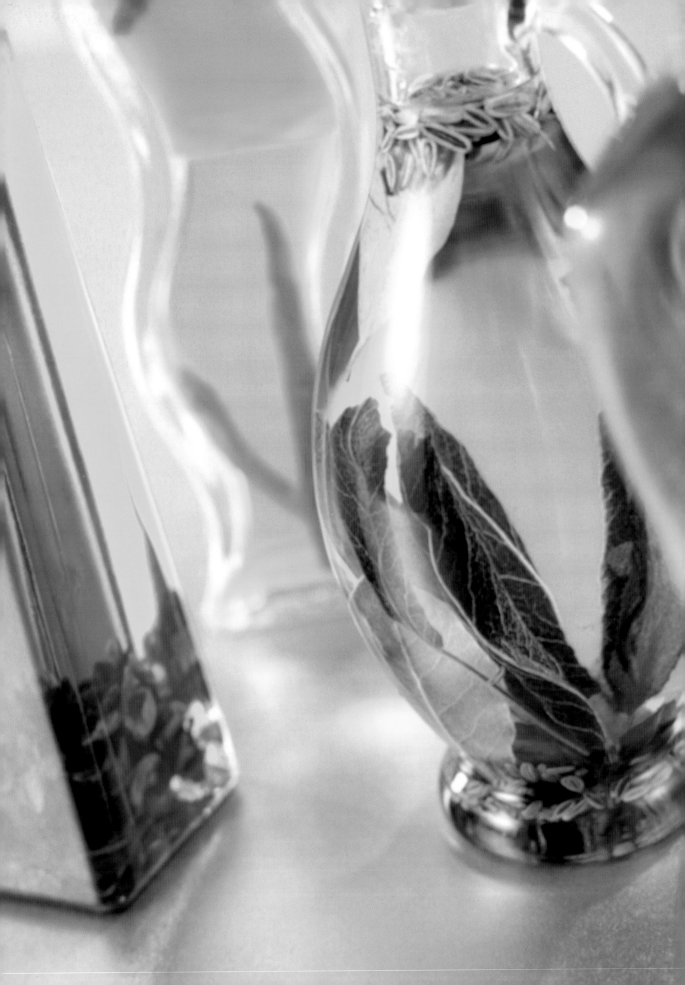

Virgin Olive Oil and Other Essential Fatty Acids

When you need to use oils in cooking (for stir-frying or grilling) or in salad dressings, always choose cold-pressed virgin olive or sunflower oils. These are monounsaturated and polyunsaturated fats – in contrast to saturated fats such as butter, cream and cheese – and these types of fat have a protective effect on both the heart and the circulatory system, discouraging the furring up of artery walls.

Although dietary fats should generally occupy no more than a 20 per cent share of the overall diet, some essential fatty acids are mandatory for the maintenance of optimum health and vitality. They include omega 3 fatty acids, which help guard against heart attacks and strokes. These are to be found in fish oils, linseeds, walnuts, pumpkin seeds and dark green, leafy vegetables. Omega 6 oils are also important dietary ingredients that help boost energy levels, enhance immune system functioning (helping us to resist infection), encourage optimum hormone balance and help to regulate metabolic rate (ensuring that your body processes don't become sluggish). Rich sources of omega 6 oils are corn, sesame, unrefined safflower and sunflower oils.

Low-caffeine or Caffeine-free Drinks

One of the best known alternatives to Indian tea and coffee is green tea. Naturally low in caffeine, green tea provides you with a refreshing hot drink that gives you a natural lift, without the health hazards of coffee. It's also rich in antioxidants and so supplies extra support in the fight against free radical production.

If you want to kick the caffeine habit altogether, there are a number of coffee substitutes available that can be surprisingly enjoyable alternatives to coffee and tea. These are grain-based formulas (often made from roasted barley with added flavourings such as chicory) that can be made up instantly as a hot drink, neat or with milk.

In addition, you can choose from an increasingly imaginative range of herbal or fruit teas that will energize or relax you depending on what you want at different times of the day. Where herbal blends are concerned, it is best not to restrict yourself to one

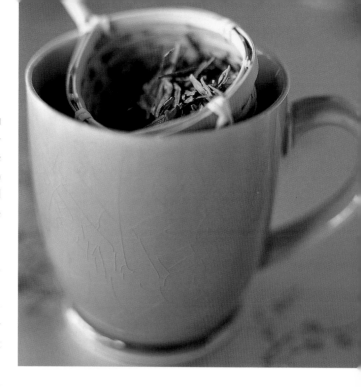

ABOVE **KICKING THE CAFFEINE HABIT WILL BE EASIER IF YOU SWITCH TO CAFFEINE-FREE DRINKS THAT YOU ENJOY.** LEFT **OPT FOR COLD-PRESSED VIRGIN OLIVE OIL WHEN CHOOSING OILS FOR SALAD DRESSINGS OR STIR-FRYING.**

blend that you drink all of the time. Apart from the inevitable risk of boredom, there is also a slight risk that your body may become sensitized to one particular herb if you overdo it for too long. For instance, while valerian in small doses can be helpful in easing headaches related to muscle tension, large doses can aggravate tension headaches.

A word of caution

When cutting caffeinated drinks out of your diet, be prepared for the onset of caffeine withdrawal. This is likely to particularly affect you if you normally drink more than six strong cups of coffee a day. The most common symptoms are a severe headache, shakiness, nausea and low energy levels. With this in mind, it can be helpful to quit the caffeine habit over a weekend so that there is more opportunity to take it easy, drink lots of water and eat light, nutritious food. In the long run, it's really going to be worth it.

WHAT YOU SEE ISN'T ALWAYS WHAT YOU GET: THE PITFALLS OF ENERGY DRINKS AND ENERGY BARS

Some of us may have been seduced into thinking that the solution to a dip in mental or physical energy during the day can be found in a can of energy-boosting soft drink. If you take a moment to look at the ingredients in these carbonated drinks, you're likely to be disappointed to find that they include a hefty proportion of sugar, as well as a liberal injection of caffeine, along with some vitamins. While they will give you an initial energy boost, the long-term energy effect is identical to the reaction described in the section on caffeinated drinks (see page 59). Be especiaclly cautious about drinking soft drinks that include guarana, as this is a form of stimulant and can have an effect similar to that of caffeine.

These drinks can bring additional problems in their wake, in the form of palpitations, difficulty falling asleep and raised anxiety levels. The 'sports' formulas unfortunately also often rely on large doses of refined sugar to impart a sensation of a temporary lift, something we have already seen does precious little for your long-term vitality.

Energy bars are also worth examining. If you look closely at the label of each bar, you will find that, although there are some variations from product to product, many of these also rely on a combination of refined cereal and sugar. Some, however, are made from a concentrated preparation of dried fruit such as apricots. While these are still fairly high in sugar, provided they include a significant amount of dietary fibre they are preferable to a bar made from refined carbohydrates. Be even more suspicious if a bar is covered in chocolate, as this will increase the sugar and saturated fat content even more.

In the main, these products are best avoided if you want sustained energy release. If you are looking for a quick snack to give you a boost, you would do far better to have a cup of green tea with a banana, a handful of unsalted and unroasted nuts or seeds (such as sunflower), or a few pieces of organic dried fruit (apricots are especially delicious and are rich in iron). Instead of reaching for a fizzy, caffeinated drink, choose one of the carbonated formulas that harness natural fruit and herbal flavourings to provide a delicious refreshing taste.

BELOW **THE SUGARS FOUND IN FRESH FRUIT ARE RELEASED INTO YOUR BODY LESS ABRUPTLY THAN REFINED SUGAR.**

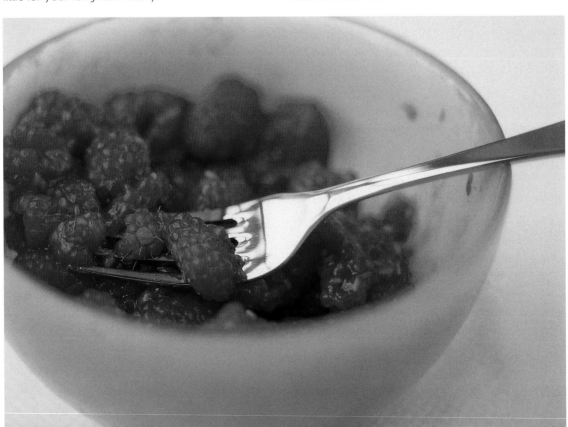

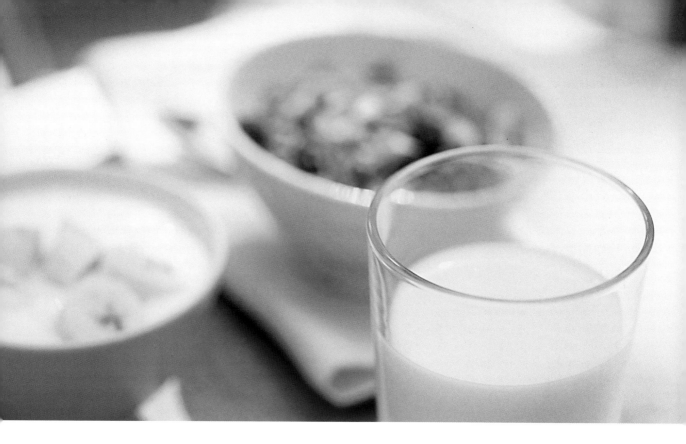

THE RE-ENERGIZING PLAN

What follows is a general guide to the foods and drinks that you should make the mainstay, of your eating plan if you want to experience high-level health and vitality on a daily basis. These are the foods and drinks that help us to summon high-level energy as and when we need it. For this advice to work well for you, you will need to apply it in the way that suits you and your lifestyle best.

For instance, you may find that you need to swap the suggestions for lunch with those for dinner occasionally. In addition, it helps to be prepared for the fact that you are bound to have days where you break the rules: either because we just can't face another day without a slice of chocolate fudge cake or because you have a night out on the town. The main thing is not to worry about it. Accept that it's healthy to break the rules infrequently, and just get back on track again the next day. Most important of all is to make sure that you always enjoy what you're eating.

ABOVE **DON'T MAKE THE MISTAKE OF SKIPPING BREAKFAST, AS THIS MEAL HELPS TO PREVENT A MIDMORNING ENERGY DIP.**

Breakfast

Never skip breakfast: eating breakfast is the most certain way of ensuring you don't hit a severe energy slump later in the day. That old cliché about it being the most important meal of the day is a cliché because it's true. Choose from any of the following options, depending on your mood:

- **Homemade muesli soaked overnight in order to break down the starches. Possible ingredients include oat, rye or wheat flakes sprinkled with sunflower seeds, organic raisins, sultanas (golden raisins) or chopped, dried apricots. Soak in organic semi-skimmed milk. If you are sensitive to dairy products, substitute fruit juice for soaking**
- **Two slices of wholemeal (wholewheat) toast with a little organic butter topped with organic fruit preserve or perhaps a drizzle of wildflower honey**
- **Green or fruit tea or coffee substitute**
- **A large glass of still mineral water or filtered tap water**

Avoid:
- **Sweetened breakfast cereals made from refined grains**
- **Fatty, fried breakfasts such as bacon and sausages**
- **Strong coffee or tea**
- **Missing breakfast**

Mid-morning

- A glass of mineral water with a twist of lemon or lime, or a cup of green or herbal tea
- If hunger pangs hit, have a piece of fruit or prepared raw vegetables cut into bite-size sticks. If this involves too much organization, eat an apple, pear or banana instead

Avoid:

- A strong cup of coffee
- Chocolate biscuits (cookies)
- Doughnuts

Lunch

Choose from any of the following:

- Wholemeal (wholewheat) pasta with a tasty, tomato-based sauce
- Two scrambled or poached organic, free-range eggs on wholemeal toast
- A piece of organic, free-range chicken breast with a mixed salad and dressing made from cold-pressed virgin olive or sunflower oil with vinegar or lemon juice
- A large mixed salad including avocado, steamed broccoli, spinach leaves, grated carrot, watercress, grated red cabbage, cauliflower, lettuce, green, red and yellow peppers, mushrooms, celery, grated hard-boiled egg, spring onions or olives. For extra substance and protein, a little tuna, mackerel or cheese may be added
- A large glass of mineral water
- A cup of green or fruit tea

Avoid:

- Burgers and French fries
- Club sandwiches with lashings of bacon, cheese and mayonnaise
- 'Instant' anything that has been dehydrated, flavoured and coloured beyond recognition. As a basic rule, if the label says 'just add hot water and stir', it is best left on the shelf unopened
- Carbonated cola drinks
- Potato crisps or fried snacks that contain lots of chemical colourings or flavourings and salt
- Cakes and biscuits (cookies) that are high in refined sugar and saturated fat
- Alcohol and coffee

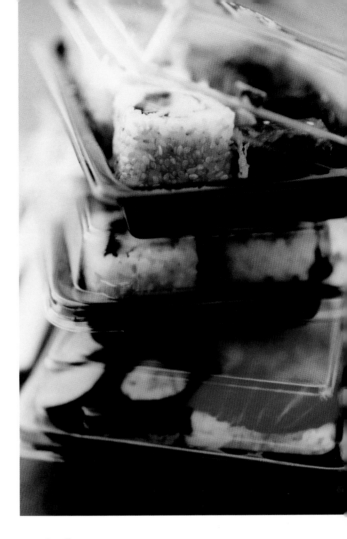

Mid-afternoon

- A large glass of water
- A cup of herbal, green or fruit tea or coffee substitute

Choose one of the following:

- A handful of unroasted, unsalted nuts, seeds and/or organic dried fruit
- A biscuit (cookie) made from organic cereal with a little unrefined sugar or honey added
- A couple of pieces of fruit

Avoid:

- A carbonated 'energy' drink
- Chocolate
- A couple of espressos and a cigarette

ABOVE KEEP LUNCH LIGHT IF YOU FACE A DEMANDING AFTERNOON WHEN YOU NEED TO STAY ALERT.

RIGHT STIR-FRYING WITH COLD-PRESSED VIRGIN OLIVE OR SUNFLOWER OIL IS A HEALTHY ALTERNATIVE TO DEEP-FRYING.

Dinner

Choose from any of the following:

- Baked potato with a generous portion of green, red and orange vegetables, plus a helping of grilled salmon or trout
- Brown rice with a vegetable curry (be sure to include lots of lentils, chickpeas and beans for texture and to provide complete protein)
- A large mixed salad as described for lunch with a portion of grilled organic, free-range chicken or a serving of fish. Dressings may be made from cold-pressed virgin olive or sunflower oil with balsamic vinegar
- A wholemeal (wholewheat) pasta dish with a tomato-based sauce to which any of the following can be added: onions, garlic, courgettes (zucchini), peppers of all colours, basil, tuna and/or prawns (shrimp)
- Stir-fried vegetables in season with shredded free-range organic chicken, prawns (shrimp), monkfish or salmon, and noodles

Plus:

- A glass of mineral water
- For dessert most nights have a generous serving of fresh fruit, bio yoghurt (i.e. 'live' yoghurt containing cultures such as acidophilus that are good for the gut) or stewed organic dried fruit
- A cup of relaxing herb tea to help wind down for the rest of the night

Avoid:

- Pizza
- Meat pies
- Heavily processed dishes that have been vacuum-packed and just need to be re-heated
- French fries with chicken nuggets or fish fingers
- Red meat
- Take-away meals
- Sticky puddings
- Ice cream

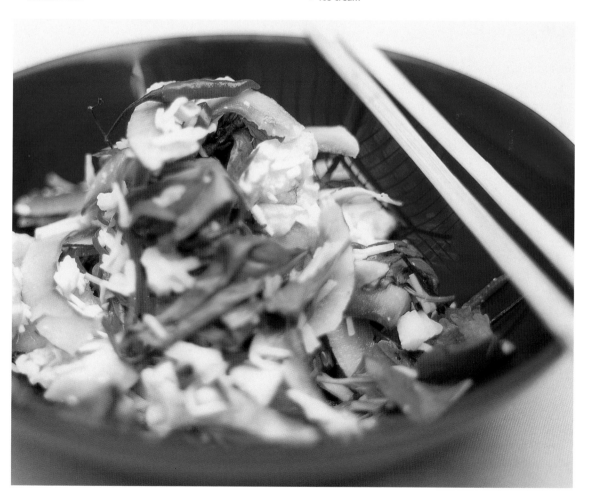

Patterns of eating for sustained energy release

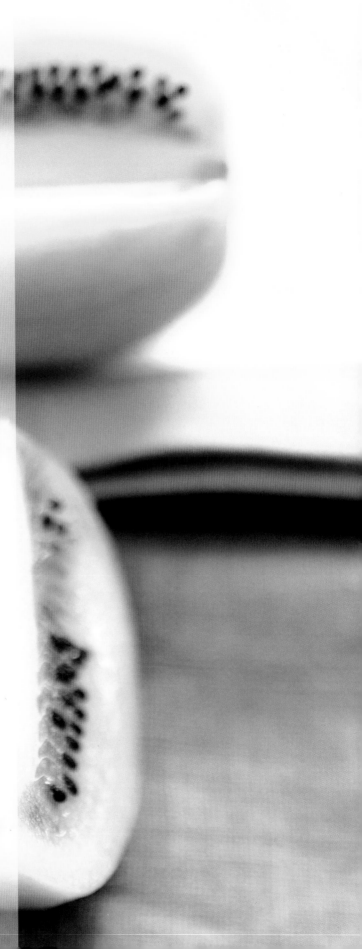

- Keep your blood sugar levels as stable as possible by taking care to have something small to eat every couple of hours or so. It needn't be anything more than a slice of wholemeal (wholewheat) bread, organic rice cake or piece of fruit. The main thing to avoid is going for hours on nothing more than a cup of coffee and slice of chocolate cake.

- Even if it feels foreign to your nature, make a point of always having a healthy breakfast. Persist until the habit becomes second nature. Breakfast will stimulate your digestive system and make it a lot less likely that that you will crave something sweet and sticky later in the day.

- If you know that you have a tendency to feel sleepy after lunch, avoid eating anything heavy or indigestible in the middle of the day, as this is sure to make things worse. Steer clear of anything fatty, fried or stodgy, opting for salads, soups, vegetables and a little fish, chicken or seafood instead.

- Try to make the basis of your daily eating pattern a healthy proportion of unrefined carbohydrates, with plenty of water, a little protein and a modest amount of dietary fat, avoiding sources of saturated fat and accenting omega 6 and omega 3 essential fatty acids instead.

- Avoid eating on the run. You need time to relax if you're going to derive maximum benefit from what you eat, so don't eat at your desk while working or simply grab a sandwich as you run to the next appointment. Take the time to make the food you are putting into your mouth a meal, rather than simply fuel to be ingested as quickly as possible.

- Don't feel guilty if you fall off the wagon from time to time. Just concentrate on bringing things back into line the following day. After all, rules are inevitably going to be broken every now and then – it's part of the fabric of life.

NUTRITIONAL QUICK-FIXES: CAFFEINE-FREE ENERGY BOOSTERS

Apart from concentrating on high-energy foods that provide you with a steady and sustained energy release, you can also occasionally make use of freshly prepared fruit smoothies to give you a much-needed energy kickstart at times when you feel that you are flagging. There are a number of important basic advantages to turning to these fresh fruit drinks when you are under pressure, rather than relying on the caffeine and refined sugar 'fixes' described above. They include the following:

- Although fruit contains its own form of sugar known as fructose, its effect on the body is less likely to give you the violent sugar 'rush' that comes as a result of ingesting large amounts of glucose (refined sugar). Processed, carbonated, sweetened colas, on the other hand, provide only 'empty' calories in the form of a hefty serving of glucose. In other words, you use energy and nutrients in order to process this sugar, but are given nothing of nutritional value in return.

- Fruit not only provides you with natural sweetness to help counteract sugar cravings, but also contains important nutrients such as antioxidant vitamins that give our immune systems a natural boost. Juices that are made by using a blender also provide a healthy amount of dietary fibre (some juicers unfortunately remove this), benefiting your digestive system greatly.

- The soluble fibre in freshly made smoothies ensures that fructose doesn't enter your bloodstream too rapidly. This is thanks to the way in which the fibre acts as a nutritional 'buffer', slowing the release of fructose into the system.

The following are some suggestions of simple combinations of fruit smoothies. Use these as a basis for experiment – you are sure to discover some favourite flavour combinations of your own.

LEFT AND RIGHT **KIWI FRUIT ARE A DELICIOUS SOURCE OF VITAMIN C, WHILE STRAWBERRIES ARE RICH IN POTASSIUM.**

Banana Smoothie

Put 1 cup (250 ml) of natural bio ('live') yoghurt, a large ripe banana, 1 teaspoon clear organic honey and a few drops of vanilla essence (extract) to taste in a blender. Process until smooth. Replace the yoghurt with milk for a less thick consistency.

Apricot Smoothie

Blend 6 sweet fresh or organic dried apricots (soaked overnight to soften) with 1½ cups (375 ml) natural bio yoghurt. Add a dash of honey if necessary to taste. Add milk to taste to lighten the texture.

Energy-busting Smoothie

Put 1 cup (250 ml) organic, semi-skimmed milk, 3 or 4 sweet strawberries or a handful of chopped, peeled ripe peach, ½ soft banana and a dash of honey in a blender. Process until smooth and thick.

QUICK NUTRITIONAL HINTS FOR THREE BASIC ENERGY TYPES

While the advice given above is generally suitable for most people, you may have discovered that you fit into one of the three energy profiles described in chapter 1 (pages 24–27). If so, here is some specially tailored nutritional advice that will help you to make even further progress in re-energizing your life.

Vata/Phosphorus Energy Type

Foods to Choose Freely

- Warming, thick vegetable-based soups
- Chunky casseroles containing small quantities of protein
- Pasta dishes
- Avocados
- Bananas
- Cherries
- Mangoes
- Dairy foods
- Cooked, warming vegetable dishes
- Spicy dishes including any of the following warming flavours: mustard, black pepper, cinnamon, ginger, cloves

Eat Infrequently or in Small Quantities

- Iced or frozen foods
- Watery foods (e.g. watermelon and cucumber)
- Apples
- Pears
- Cranberries
- Sprouts
- Convenience foods (i.e. anything dehydrated or artificially coloured or flavoured)
- Alcohol

Pitta/Nux Vomica Energy Type

Foods to Choose Freely

- Cooling, watery salad vegetables (e.g. cucumber)
- Milk
- Mild cheeses (e.g. Jarlsberg or Edam)
- Grapes
- Melons
- Apples
- Sweet, ripe oranges
- Green vegetables
- Cauliflower
- Fresh peas
- Digestive-balancing spices and herbs, including coriander, cumin, fennel, mint, turmeric

Eat Infrequently or in Small Quantities

- Red meat
- Alcohol
- Excessively spicy, warming foods
- Salty foods
- Fried or fatty 'junk' foods
- Sour foods such as grapefruit or blueberries
- Onions
- Sour cream or yoghurt

Kapha/Calc Carb Energy Type

Foods to Choose Freely

- Light, easily digested, dry-textured foods
- Salads
- Fresh vegetables
- Apples
- Pears
- Fish
- Pulses
- Most spices, but especially cayenne, ginger, pepper, garlic

Eat Infrequently or in Small Quantities

- Sweet foods such as desserts and ice cream
- Dairy products
- Salty foods
- Fried foods
- Frozen foods
- Bananas
- Melons
- Sweet potatoes
- Avocados

RIGHT ALWAYS REMEMBER THAT MEALTIMES SHOULD IDEALLY BE AS PLEASURABLE, BALANCED AND RELAXED AS POSSIBLE IF YOU ARE TO DRAW THE FULL BENEFITS OF THE EXPERIENCE OF EATING. IN OTHER WORDS, THERE IS MORE TO FOOD THAN SIMPLY FUELLING UP.

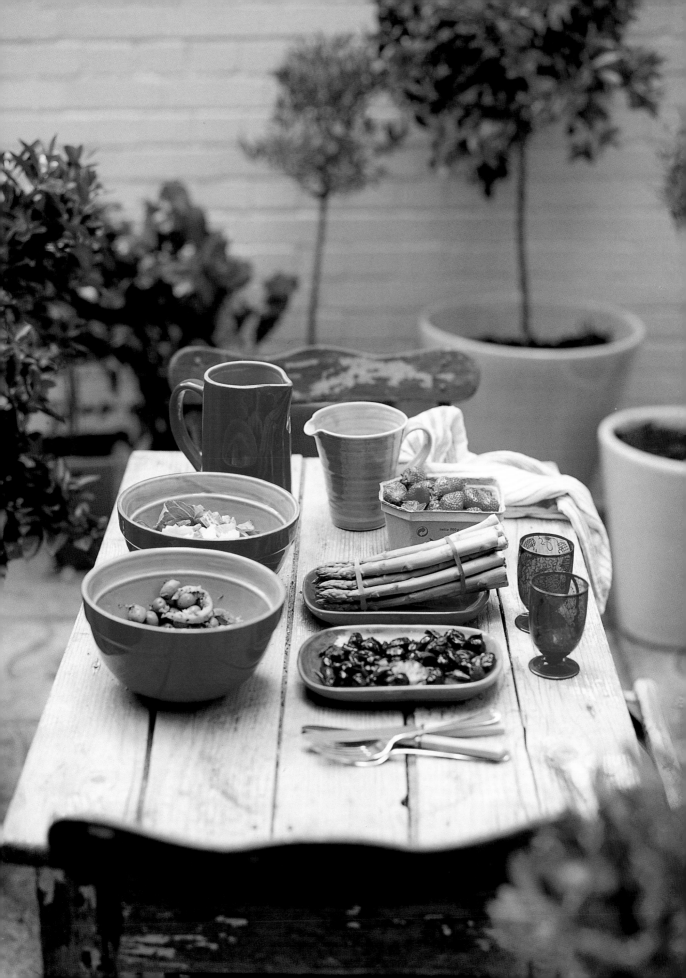

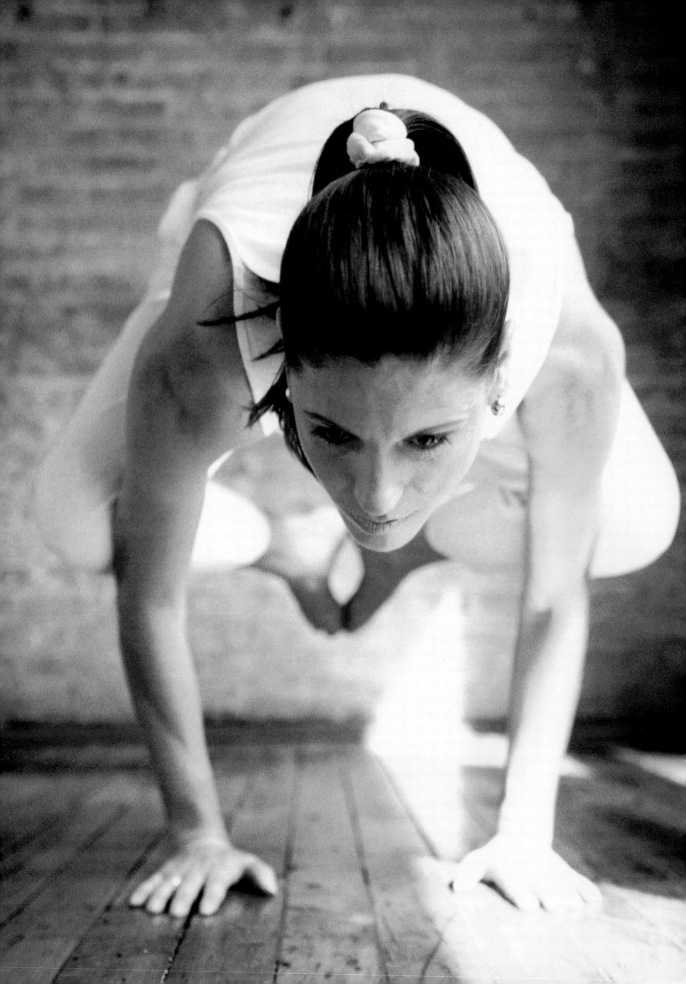

4 Body stamina

There can't be many of us left who remain completely unaware of the all-round benefits of becoming more physically fit. Glossy magazines, gym advertisements and television programmes focusing on health and fitness all throw images of well-toned bodies at us with relentless regularity. While this is fine, as getting into physical shape has undoubted health benefits, the types of exercise and systems of movement outlined in this chapter will take us beyond a narrow concentration on ensuring that our bodies are knocked into better shape.

While every exercise system explained in this section undoubtedly has an impact on improving muscle strength, overall stamina and flexibility, and generally creating a leaner body shape through encouraging healthier postural habits, each one also brings significant benefits in its wake that enhance these physical improvements. These systems of movement have a well-established track record, with regular practitioners of each discipline testifying to the profound effects that are recognized to benefit the mind, emotions and body. As all of the systems are known to encourage optimum mental, emotional and physical balance, this makes any of these exercise options a hugely appropriate choice if you want to manage negative stress effectively.

LEFT IF YOU'RE A NEWCOMER TO YOGA, JOIN A CLASS THAT IS SUPERVISED BY A FULLY QUALIFIED PRACTITIONER.

What is more to the point is that appropriate systems of physical movement can have a significant role to play in balancing your energy levels. They gently lift a chronically low level of vitality and reduce nervous energy in those of us who find it difficult to switch off and relax when we need to.

Tell-tale signs of low vitality

Low vitality generally doesn't suddenly spring upon you with no warning, although sometimes this can seem to be the case. One moment you think that you are travelling along through life relatively smoothly, then the next you realize that your daily actions seem plagued with a general malaise. Usually, though, a feeling of low vitality creeps up on you in a slow and insidious fashion. But don't despair. There are several tell-tale signs of low vitality that warn you something is amiss in time to head it off:

- **Generalized tension and aches and pains**
- **Recurrent minor infections**
- **Mood swings**
- **Lack of focus**
- **Poor motivation**
- **Disturbed, fitful sleep**

THE NEED FOR MOVEMENT

Movement is intrinsic to balanced energy production. The analogy of a high-performance car has already been used in the nutrition chapter to explain why your body needs the best-quality food in order to perform to its optimum capacity. But that is only half of the story. Even if you take the care to put the best grade fuel in your car, leaving it idle for extended periods of time will still mean that the battery goes flat in no time at all and mechanical parts will begin to seize up. In principle, the same is true of your body, sometimes painfully so.

Your body's joints and muscles are structures that positively benefit from appropriate, challenging physical activity. When you stop using your muscles for any reason – for instance, after a period of bed rest following surgery or a long illness – you are likely to be shocked by the speed at which you lose muscle strength and bulk. The resulting wobbliness and weakness can make you feel distressingly weary and drained. It can also come as a surprise that it takes you significantly longer proportionately to rebuild your muscle strength than it did to lose it in the first place. Of course, the examples given above are extreme cases; however, if you contemplate the

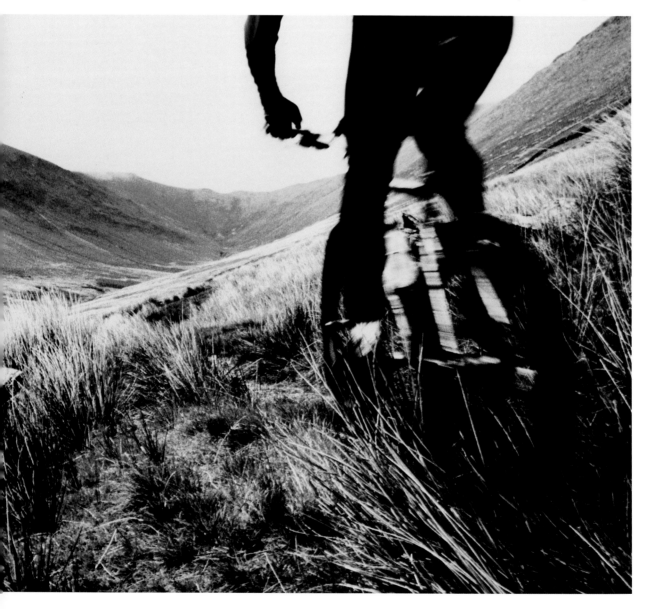

subtle, undermining effects of having long-neglected, under-used muscles on your overall sense of vitality, strength and stamina, you can see that this is something to guard against.

Your muscles also play an additional centrally important role in the functioning of your immune system. This is in relation to the movement of lymphatic fluid through your lymph vessels and lymph nodes. The lymphatic system as a whole works as a fundamental part of your immune system, filtering out and eliminating toxins and, as a result, helping the body to fight infection.

For all of this to work as smoothly and efficiently as possible, you are dependent on the unobstructed, flowing movement of lymphatic fluid. The lymphatic system, unlike the circulatory system, doesn't have a central pump like the heart to get the fluid moving on its way. This means that your body is heavily dependent on the contraction and relaxation of the large muscle groups of the arms and legs to keep lymphatic fluid flowing efficiently and smoothly. When you take this into account, it becomes easy to see how a seriously sedentary lifestyle does nothing to stimulate your lymphatic system, and this can contribute to your feeling generally lacklustre and below par most of the time.

If you're physically inactive, there's also a fighting chance that you are losing out on optimum oxygen absorption through breathing less than efficiently. Breathing is classed as an involuntary reflex – in other words, we don't have to think about it consciously to make it happen. Many of us simply leave it to take care of itself. Unfortunately, this lack of awareness can bring with it a host of problems. These are explored in 'Breathing for energy' on page 79.

Improved vitality is not the only positive outcome of stimulating the efficient movement of lymphatic fluid. There are also cosmetic benefits, which bring their own rewards in terms of self-esteem. These include generally clearer, brighter skin and a reduced tendency to develop cellulite.

LEFT **DON'T FORGET THAT CYCLING NEED NOT BE LIMITED TO THE OUTDOORS. YOU CAN ALSO BENEFIT FROM USING A STATIONARY EXERCISE BIKE INDOORS IN ANY FREE TIME.**

THE PRICE WE PAY FOR A SEDENTARY LIFESTYLE

Apart from the drawbacks already mentioned, there are more general, subtle problems that tend to follow from turning into a couch potato. They can include any of the following:

Physical Tension

Many of us may be draining ourselves of energy on a daily basis by holding tension in our muscles and joints without even being aware of doing so. You can discover at first hand just how tiring it can be to hold your muscles in a state of tension by carrying out the following simple exercise.

Clench your hand in a fist, tensing the muscles of the forearm and upper arm at the same time. Breathe normally, holding the arm in this position for a minute or two, then relax the limb completely. You should find that letting go and relaxing the tension will have resulted in a feeling of great relief. Now imagine holding that sort of tension on a low-grade level in other muscle groups (e.g. the face, scalp, shoulders and back) without even being aware of it.

By concentrating on systems of exercise and movement that focus on relaxing and gently stretching specific muscle groups, such as yoga, t'ai chi and Pilates, you allow yourself the chance to relearn your postural habits. Once you are aware of where you are holding tension, and consciously let go, you should experience steadily enhanced energy levels, as well as greater emotional balance and mental clarity and focus.

Mood Swings

If you often feel briefly low or 'blue' for no particular reason, you should benefit from the mood-balancing effect of regular, aerobic exercise that conditions your heart and lungs. Power walking, cycling, dancing or running on a regular basis (three or four 45-minute sessions a week may be all you need) provides the benefit of enhanced secretion of those naturally occurring, feel-good chemicals known as endorphins.

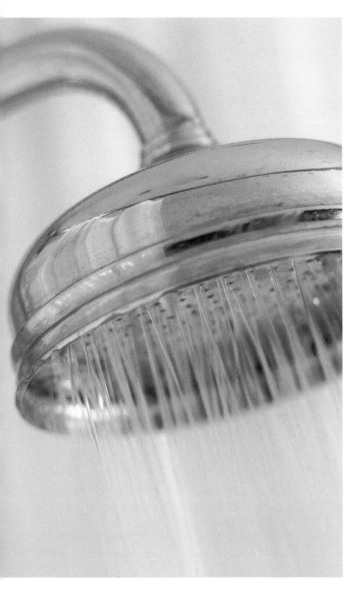

Poor Skin Tone and Texture

Sluggish lymphatic fluid movement (see page 77) can result in poor skin tone and texture. Cellulite – the bumpy, 'orange peel' skin that can form on upper arms, buttocks and thighs – is thought to be a sign of the stagnant condition of the affected tissues. This is considered to be the end result of an established state of poor circulatory function combined with a sluggish flow of lymphatic fluid.

In addition to being a cosmetic blight, cellulite is thought to indicate that your system isn't eliminating toxic wastes from your tissues as efficiently as it should. If you do have problems with established cellulite, you may also find you suffer from recurrent fatigue due to a generally sluggish system.

Regular exercise that gets your major muscle groups moving will help your lymphatic system tremendously and give you the best chance of putting a cellulite-busting plan into action. You should also start implementing the following if you want to say good-bye to that cellulite:

- **Dry skin brushing every day has a stimulating effect on the movement of lymphatic fluid. Use a long-handled natural-bristle brush, making long, sweeping strokes over the body before showering. Avoid brushing any areas of broken, sore or inflamed skin.**

- **Lengthy, overhot baths are not advisable, as they encourage sagging and blotchy skin. Use moderately warm water instead, and make sure that you don't soak in the water for too long.**

- **Try a quick burst of cold water at the end of a warm shower. This simple hydrotherapy technique can help to kick-start your system if you feel sluggish or muzzy-headed, and increases micro-circulation of the skin.**

- **Eliminate or cut down on any items in your diet that are known to contribute to cellulite. These include tea, coffee, alcohol, carbonated drinks, saturated fats and anything with a high sugar content. Concentrate instead on lots of filtered water, fruit and herbal teas, fresh fruit, vegetables and fibre-rich foods (to avoid constipation).**

These appear to be responsible for the natural 'high' that typically follows sustained bouts of aerobic activity. Engaging in regular aerobic exercise is one of the best ways to attain emotional balance.

There are other psychological benefits that come from enjoying regular physical movement. Your self-confidence and self-esteem should grow from having a body that moves freely and with suppleness, strength and ease. This in itself is a huge mental and emotional energy booster and is nothing whatsoever to do with having the 'perfect' body.

ABOVE **YOUR SHOWER CAN ACT AS A SIMPLE HYDROTHERAPY TREATMENT IN LIEU OF MORE SOPHISTICATED ONES.**

Breathing for energy

Most of us take breathing for granted. After all, you don't have to think consciously about it, yet you still breathe in and out seemingly without effort. Unfortunately, you tend to slip into the habit of using a small proportion of your overall breathing capacity, and this can be further diminished if you become tense and anxious. Upper-body tension leads you to breathe in an increasingly shallow and rapid manner, so that you feel even more edgy and short-fused. Unsurprisingly, breathing in this way for any length of time also makes you feel muzzy-headed and lethargic, and you start to yawn frequently in order to redress the oxygen/carbon dioxide imbalance.

The good news is that there are simple breathing techniques for maximizing oxygen uptake that you can call on whenever you feel tired, lacking in sparkle or tense. These exercises are an invaluable way of clearing the mind and recharging your energy batteries. If you suffer from any medical problems, seek professional advice before using any breathing techniques.

Alternate nostril breathing

1 **Bend the three middle fingers of your right hand so that they rest against the palm of that hand, leaving the thumb and little finger extended.**
2 **Rest your thumb lightly against your right nostril, while breathing in for a count of four through your left nostril.**
3 **Close both nostrils for a count of four by keeping your thumb in position and resting your little finger on your left nostril.**
4 **Remove your thumb, and breathe out through your right nostril for a count of four.**
5 **Pause for a moment before completing the cycle by breathing in through the right nostril first.**
6 **Repeat the exercise four times on each side to give your body a wake-up call and sharpen your mind.**

Ujjayi breathing

Sometimes referred to as 'fire breathing', this is a basic technique used in ashtanga yoga to relax you and to balance energy levels in the body.

1 **Sit in quiet, peaceful surroundings that allow you to concentrate undisturbed on what you are doing.**

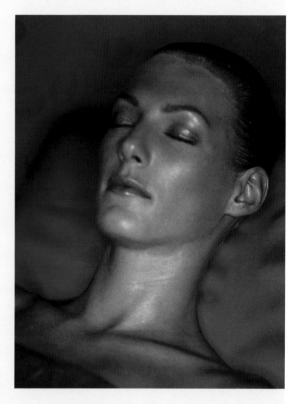

2 **Take a full breath while focusing on tightening the muscles around your throat. If you are doing this correctly, you should hear a soft, hissing sound as you breathe in.**
3 **Breathe out gently, still focusing on keeping the muscles tight around your throat. This should result in a sound that is rather similar to the noise made by *Star Wars*' Darth Vader behind his mask.**
4 **Take six breaths in this way before having a rest. Once you are familiar with how it should feel and sound, this cycle of six breaths can be done four times. Make sure that you always take a break between each repetition.**

ENERGY-BALANCING SYSTEMS OF MOVEMENT

This is a brief tour of some of the most thoroughly road-tested forms of movement that have a reputation for encouraging optimum balance of mental, emotional and physical energy.

Yoga

The acknowledged benefits of regular yoga practice are impressively wide-ranging. Enhanced ability to relax, higher energy levels, greater all-round stamina, improved muscle strength and increased flexibility and freedom from stiffness are just some of the known positive changes that are experienced as a result of becoming adept at practising yoga.

Although often referred to as one thing, it helps to bear in mind that there are a number of different approaches to yoga that vary in their intensity, pace and overall objectives. Hatha yoga is generally the best choice for beginners who want to find an effective way to start improving muscle strength, stamina, flexibility and learn simple but powerful breathing techniques to revitalize or calm themselves.

Ashtanga or 'power' yoga has generated a great deal of attention over the past few years as a result of celebrity interest and enthusiasm. This is unlikely to be a suitable first choice for the unfit, however, as it's extremely physically challenging. On the other hand,

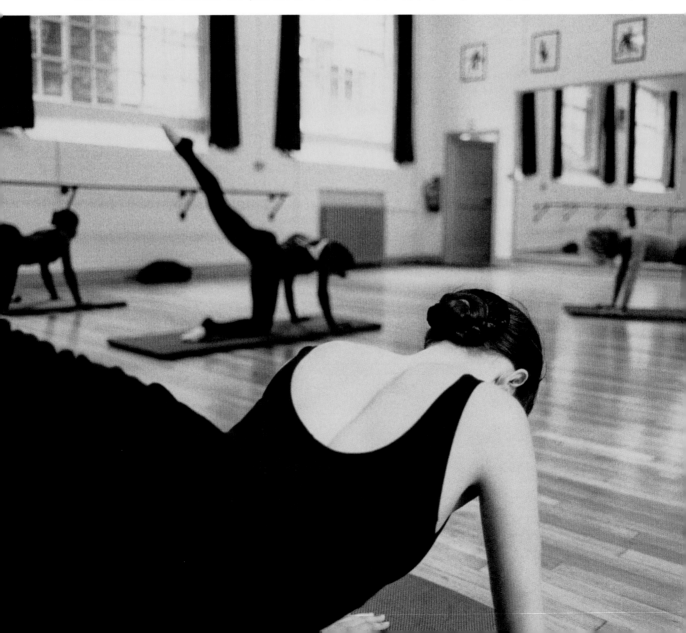

if you're generally physically fit and want to find a system of movement that helps to harmonize both mind and body, while enabling you to develop a supple, stronger, leaner body, ashtanga yoga may well be the perfect one to explore.

Yoga provides a very refreshing contrast to the punishing, competitive exercise classes that became so popular during the 1980s. In yoga, there is no encouragement of a 'no pain, no gain' approach. Basically, if it hurts you don't do it, as this is a sure sign that there is a risk of injury. Also, in yoga class, you are not in competition with anyone else – you are just looking for progression in yourself.

Whichever form of yoga you want to pursue, beginners should always make a point of going to classes run by trained practitioners in order to learn how to perform the postures as accurately as possible. This is extremely important, for maximum benefit will only be obtained from the poses if you execute them correctly. The safety issue is also one you should never neglect. Yoga practice is very challenging. You could inadvertently hurt yourself if you repeatedly practise a posture incorrectly or try to tackle an advanced pose too soon.

This is where the tuition and advice of a fully trained teacher comes in, as he or she should be able to assess which postures are suitable for each pupil's level of expertise. The experience and training of a qualified practitioner are vital to good yoga practice. If you have any specific health problems (such as rheumatoid arthritis or high blood pressure), always mention this to the teacher before you start the class. For menstruating women, the stage of your cycle may be relevant to practising some inverted postures, as some of these should be avoided just before or during a period. Once the basic postures are familiar, it can be helpful to back up the work done in class by using a yoga video at home, but do make sure that you are proficient at the exercises before you venture out on your own.

LEFT **IT'S NEVER TOO LATE TO BECOME PHYSICALLY FIT; YOU JUST NEED TO FIND A SYSTEM OF MOVEMENT THAT SUITS YOUR PERSONALITY. YOU MAY FIND THAT YOU GET MAXIMUM BENEFIT FROM A STRETCHING CLASS.**

Pilates

An ideal system of precise movements, Pilates classes should be considered if you want to find an exercise method that helps to reduce the negative effects of mental, emotional and physical stress without placing undue strain on your body. You will also be benefiting from a fitness programme that promotes a taller, leaner body shape and encourages supple muscles and stronger joints.

The Pilates system was initially developed as a physiotherapeutic system in the 1920s, but it has gained significant popularity in the past decade or so. The exercises involve the execution of controlled, precise movements that are designed to work in an intense way on isolated muscle groups separately. Although the movements in themselves may be small, they are often held for quite a long time, with the result that you should feel that you've worked quite hard after a class.

Pilates classes focus on building a point of core stability in the torso (roughly extending from the base of the ribcage to the area between the hip bones). Some of the movements are performed standing upright, while others are carried out lying on an exercise mat. When you go to a class, some gyms make use of specialized Pilates equipment.

The benefits that come from regular practice of Pilates are impressively varied. They can include increased flexibility, improved emotional and mental balance, leaner, longer muscles, tighter muscle tone and better-aligned posture. As these movements require a great deal of concentration in order to do them as precisely and correctly as possible, while at the same time focusing on co-ordinating breathing steadily and deeply, regular practice of Pilates can have a dramatic effect on reducing the negative effects of stress. As a result, it may also have a beneficial effect on lowering blood pressure and slowing the heart rate.

It really is imperative that you attend a class given by a fully trained practitioner in order to familiarize yourself with what is involved in the exercises. Ideally, classes should be small enough to allow the teacher to give individual attention when it's needed.

T'ai Chi

The pedigree of t'ai chi is well established, as this system of gentle, coordinated movement was developed in the Far East as a martial art more than 1,000 years ago. It is believed that regular practice of the flowing movements combined with breathing exercises that make up t'ai chi can create an enhanced state of mental clarity and emotional tranquillity, boost confidence and increase muscle tone and basic physical coordination. T'ai chi is designed to stimulate greater harmony between mind, emotions and body, while also having an impressive effect on balancing energy levels.

This can certainly be a beneficial system of movement if you feel constantly hyped up or if you feel as though you're wading through treacle most of the time because of a constant feeling of fatigue. After all, either of these opposite ends of the spectrum can be triggered by the same problem: unbalanced energy levels. If t'ai chi appeals to you, it can provide the vital key you need to unlock stagnant energy streams so that they are free to flow smoothly and harmoniously once again.

In a t'ai chi class, you will be taught how to execute a series of controlled, graceful, flowing movements while keeping conscious control of your breathing. It is claimed that regular practice of t'ai chi brings a balanced flow of energy in the body, while also relaxing the muscles and improving circulation.

Acknowledged benefits of regular practice include stronger, more flexible joints, flexible, well-toned muscles, improved posture and a greater sense of physical balance and coordination. If you suffer from stress-related problems such as anxiety, you should consider taking up t'ai chi because of the emphasis that is placed on the importance of regulating the breath. This is especially helpful if you tend to hyperventilate when you feel stressed. Developing a conscious awareness of how you breathe in order to induce a more tranquil mental and emotional state can give you an important practical tool to use whenever you feel under pressure.

As with yoga, it's important to make a point of attending a class with a fully trained and qualified practitioner in order to learn how to do the basic movements correctly. Practising any system of postures incorrectly will severely diminish the potential benefits to be gained from it.

Chi Gong

The discipline of chi gong is thought to be one of the most relaxing, stress-reducing and energy-balancing systems of movement available to us. It can be especially helpful if you feel your mental energy is flagging, with the resulting poor concentration levels. Regular practice of chi gong can help you to focus mentally, so that you can achieve and sustain clarity of mind and concentration when you need it most.

In common with all of the systems of movement mentioned previously, chi gong teaches you how to breathe regularly and deeply in coordination with a series of flowing movements that are performed slowly and repetitively. As you execute all these movements, you are encouraged to focus the mind so that you're not distracted by intruding thoughts during your practice of chi gong. Once the movements become more familiar, you should find that your overall energy levels become more balanced, your general health improves and you fight off minor infections more effectively. Chi gong appears to have a beneficial effect on the performance of the body's immune system. In addition, physical co-ordination and stamina should also benefit from regular practice.

Chi gong may be taught on a one-to-one basis by a traditional Chinese practitioner, or it may be possible to attend a small class in your local area. Don't attempt to teach yourself from a book. It's unlikely that you will receive maximum benefit unless you're executing this system of movement as correctly as possible, and you may injure yourself unless you know exactly what you are doing.

RIGHT **THE ORIENTAL PRACTICES OF T'AI CHI AND CHI GONG ARE GRACEFUL, CALMING AND REBALANCING SYSTEMS OF MOVEMENT THAT HELP YOU TO FOCUS YOUR MIND, AS WELL AS IMPROVING GENERAL PHYSICAL COORDINATION.**

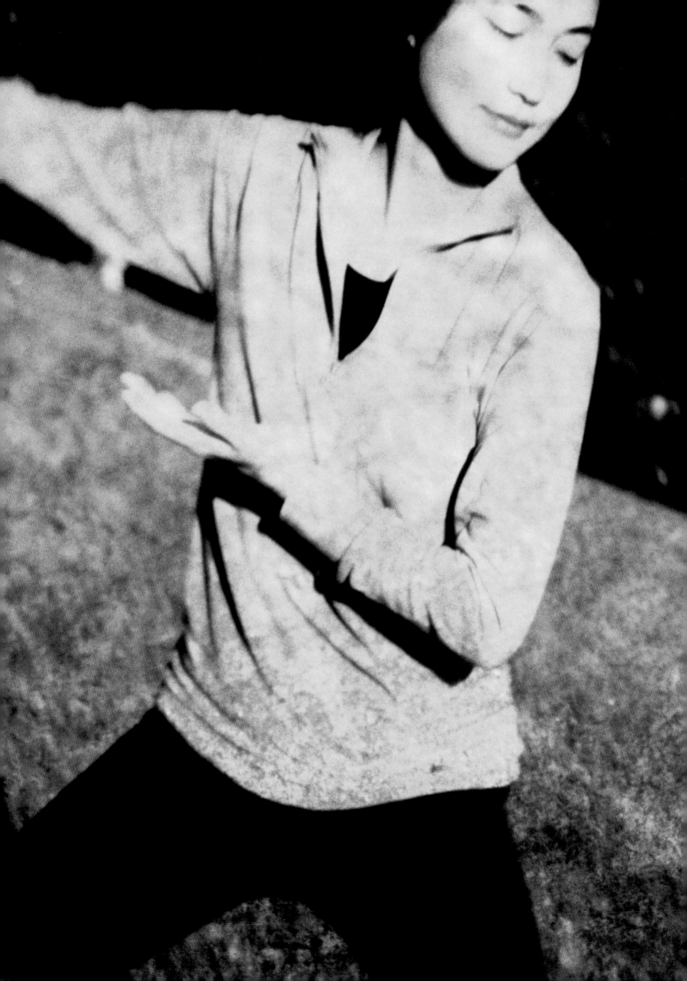

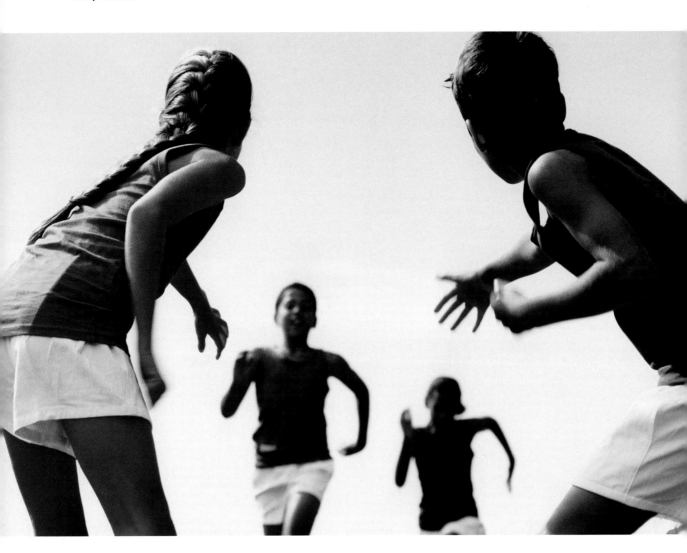

WORKABLE EXERCISE GOALS FOR COUCH POTATOES

This section is written with the absolute beginner in mind. It deliberately takes into account the usual pitfalls that entrap the newcomer to physical fitness at an early stage. By taking a very basic, practical approach to setting realistic goals at the outset, there's a far greater chance that you will continue to build on this basic framework in a way that encourages you to make physical fitness a part of your daily routine.

Ruthless Realism

The greatest obstacle to making a physical fitness programme part of your daily life is usually the tendency to be overambitious. If you haven't exercised

ABOVE **DON'T BE PUT OFF EXERCISING IF YOU DIDN'T ENJOY TEAM SPORTS AS A CHILD. JUST CHOOSE WHAT SUITS YOUR TEMPERAMENT AND FITNESS LEVEL AS AN ADULT.**

before, you may often feel that you have to make an outright onslaught in order to make up for lost time. In reality, this is likely to cause you to fall at the first hurdle rather than sustain commitment in the long term. Instead, you need to work out how much time you realistically have available to you, and work within those boundaries, however small they may be.

The same is true of your physical capabilities, as it would be foolish to think that you're going to be able to run a half-marathon after a few weeks of training if you're starting from the baseline of being very unfit. If you start slowly, realistically and steadily, however, expanding the commitment steadily and organically, you are far more likely to find this builds into a plan for life. Avoid the temptation to go for the quick fix. Establishing long-term goals will promote a much greater chance of success.

Temperament and Taste

Many of us will have been through the negative experience of being swept along by the latest fitness fad just because it's fashionable, overlooking the fact that it really doesn't suit us. When this happens, of course, it's only a matter of time before you find a host of excuses to duck out of the next class. Whatever form of exercise you choose to take up, it must be fun, enjoyable and suit your personality. After all, there's little point in gritting your teeth and tolerating a t'ai chi class if you're bored out of your mind. On the other hand, it can be helpful to give something slightly unusual a chance, as you may find that you respond really well to something that wouldn't necessarily have been an obvious choice.

Loner or Party Person?

You will probably already have noticed that most of the systems of movement described above require you to make the time and commitment to attend a class regularly in order to make sure that you're performing the exercises correctly. This is great if you prefer the conviviality of a class atmosphere, and, if you do feel this way, you are probably going to benefit from the focus that a class can give. On the other hand, it may suit you better to exercise at home using a video, especially if time is really tight or you prefer to exercise at times that suit your schedule. If this is the case, it's essential that you attend a class long enough to ensure that you're able to perform the movements correctly. From this point, you are free to progress at your own pace.

Don't Look Back

Even if you have a history of not being naturally sporty or were unfit as a child, don't be put off. Thankfully, all of the systems of exercise mentioned

here are noncompetitive, as each one can be applied to suit individual needs. You need only measure your progress against your own development – anyone else's is irrelevant. Perhaps you have been alienated by the 'going for the burn' approach that dominated the fitness ethos of the 1980s. Although challenging, none of the systems of movement we are concerned with in this chapter should ever cause pain or injury. Quite the reverse is true. You should feel revitalized, balanced, clear-headed and relaxed after a session.

Options for problem areas

This is a checklist of some of the most suitable systems of movement to consider if you suffer from any of the following physical limitations:

Generalized stiffness and restricted range of flexibility

- **Yoga**
- **Pilates**
- **T'ai chi**

Tight, tense clenched muscles

- **Chi gong**
- **T'ai chi**
- **Yoga**
- **Pilates**
- **Relaxation techniques**

Poor aerobic fitness

- **Cycling**
- **Running**
- **Skipping**
- **Dancing**
- **Swimming**
- **Power walking**
- **Gym work with specialized machines to build cardiovascular fitness**

TAILORING EXERCISE PLANS TO YOUR ENERGY PROFILE

All of the generalized suggestions given so far still apply when making a choice regarding the sort of exercise system that you take up in order to improve your baseline levels of energy and vitality. However, the following perspective is designed to provide additional information to help you to choose the form of physical movement that is going to suit your individual constitutional type best.

Vata/Phosphorus Energy Profile

Motivation can be a real problem for this energy type, but for different reasons from the general sluggishness experienced by the kapha/calc carb type (see opposite). If you have a vata/phosphorus profile, you will have a tendency to burn up food easily. This often results in a slim build, which removes the motivation of needing to get into physical shape. This constitutional type can also have a problem with staying power, with the result that fitness fads can be taken up with huge enthusiasm for a short time, only to be abandoned when newer and apparently more interesting diversions come along.

The ideal type of exercise for people with a vata/phosphorus profile is one that encourages a sense of being grounded, focused and balanced. Suitable choices could include any of the following:

- **Walking**
- **Yoga**
- **T'ai chi**
- **Cycling**
- **Dancing**
- **Pilates**

Pitta/Nux Vomica Energy Profile

A general fitness regime that has a soothing, calming effect should be the main priority for this energy type. Anything that is overly competitive should be avoided, as this element of pressure is only likely to cause more tension for anyone with a pitta/nux

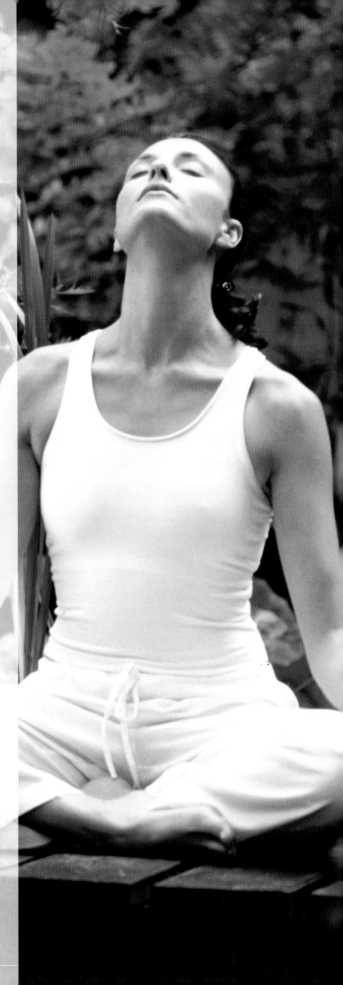

vomica profile. If this begins to happen, a new fitness programme will backfire by becoming yet another energy-draining factor in an already stressful lifestyle. Suitable, energy-balancing possibilities for pitta/nux vomica energy types include any of the following:

- Yoga
- The Alexander technique (Although this is not strictly an exercise system, this technique can help immensely in identifying postural habits which aggravate physical, mental and emotional tension.)
- T'ai chi
- Swimming

Kapha/Calc Carb Energy Profile

The key to improving the general health and vitality of this energy type is stimulation, rather than relaxation. In no other area is this more true than in the type of exercise that is likely to benefit those of us who have this underlying constitutional profile.

For kapha/calc carb energy types, the greatest obstacle to making a fitness programme work is motivation. Once energy levels start to shift in response to regular exercise, the commitment to continue will follow as the undeniable benefits of getting physical emerge. Suitable forms of exercise include:

- Brisk walking
- Running – this needs to be built up gently and very slowly if you have a history of being unfit
- Aquaerobics
- Gym work including weight training and cardiovascular workouts – under strict supervision in order to avoid injury
- Cycling
- Swimming
- Kick boxing
- Dancing

LEFT **REGULAR EXERCISE ENABLES US TO RELAX.**
BELOW **GIVE YOURSELF TIME TO RECOVER AND COOL DOWN AFTER ANY EXERCISE SESSION.**

Safety first

Whatever your energy profile, always bear the following commonsense tips in mind in order to exercise safely:

- **Never exercise on a full stomach. Allow a couple of hours at least to go by after a meal before exercising.**
- **Always avoid engaging abruptly in any system of demanding movement. Make sure that you spend plenty of time warming up cold muscles with gentle stretching movements.**
- **Never stop exercising abruptly, but always give yourself enough time to cool down and relax rather than dashing on to the next activity.**
- **It's never a good idea to take any form of exercise when feeling generally unwell, but it is especially unwise if you have a severe cold or any other viral illness that gives you a high temperature.**
- **If you experience any pain or discomfort during exercise, always stop immediately. The same is true**

of dizziness or palpitations. If any of these occur severely or frequently, seek medical advice rather than trying to break through any pain barriers.

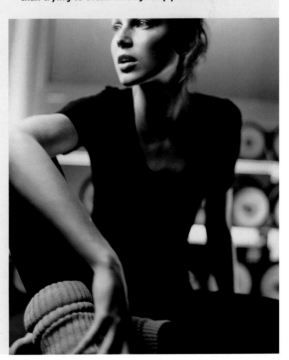

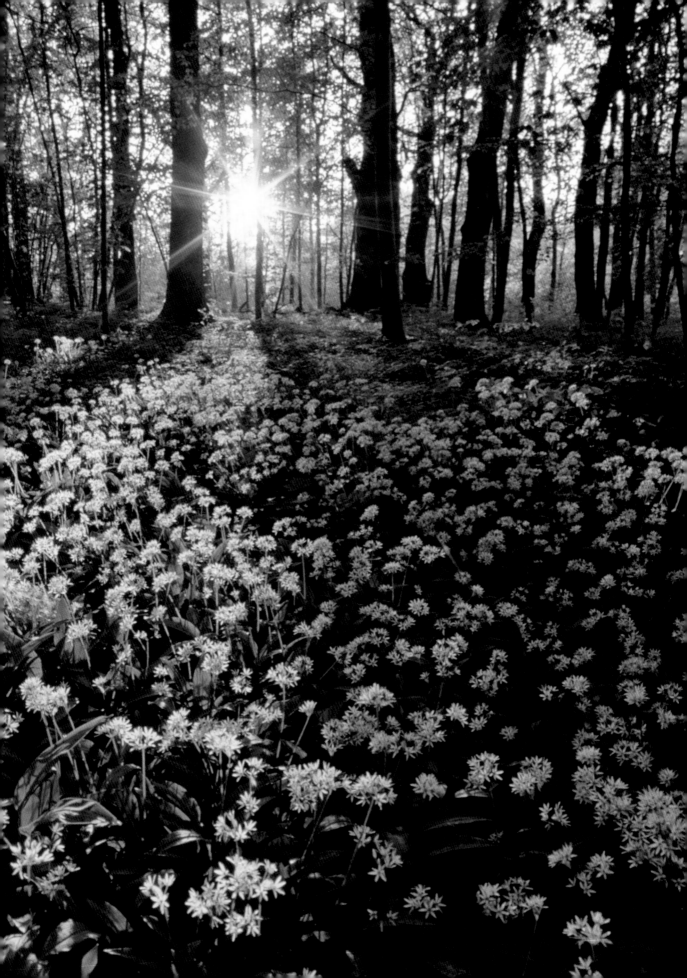

5 Sensual vitality

One of the most exciting aspects of adopting a holistic approach to healing is the way in which you begin to appreciate the important role that your immediate environment plays in stimulating and supporting optimum vitality and high-quality health. After all, you can work very hard on improving the quality of what you eat, taking care to exercise regularly and learning basic relaxation skills. If you live in an environment that is energy draining or even downright unhealthy, however, you're going to have of an more uphill task on your hands than if your surroundings are supportive of good health.

But don't worry. Creating a balanced, energy-promoting atmosphere doesn't require a huge amount of money and free time. It's just a question of being aware of the simple, practical changes that can make all the difference in helping you feel inspired rather than despondent, and energized rather than drained. Once you identify what these are – and you can be sure that they are going to be slightly different for each one of us, depending on our individual tastes and temperaments – you will be free to begin consciously to create an environment that makes you feel nurtured, invigorated and refreshed.

LEFT **IF YOU FIND A PARTICULAR PLACE OR SCENE MAKES YOU FEEL RELAXED OR PERHAPS UPLIFTED, YOU CAN CALL AN IMAGE OF THAT PLACE TO MIND WHENEVER YOU PRACTISE A VISUALIZATION EXERCISE.**

ENERGY AND OUR SURROUNDINGS

It's undeniably true that some surroundings by their very nature make us feel calm, balanced, positive and revitalized, while others can trigger feelings of gloom, uneasiness or exhaustion. Think of the difference in effect that a woodland or seaside scene can have compared to an industrial landscape. It's not just a question of the visual aspect either, for sounds, smells and air quality can all have a powerful impact on whether you feel uplifted, calm or despondent.

Individual responses also come into this equation very strongly. Some of us may find a mountain location blissfully invigorating, while others may become anxious and uncomfortable in the same atmosphere. For many, the soft green of a wooded area can feel powerfully uplifting and soothing, while others may feel enclosed and even claustrophobic. Whatever your individual instinct dictates, you should ideally make a point of recharging your energy batteries by spending free time at regular intervals in whatever surroundings make you feel refreshed.

Don't worry if you can't always find the time to travel to the place that makes you feel especially positive. If you have a vivid imagination, you can conjure up an image of that special place whenever you feel stressed or pressured. Think of it as taking a visual – or virtual – holiday.

PRACTICALITIES

You may not always be able to control your immediate environment. For instance, the choice of where you live is often more likely to be determined by job opportunities than personal preference alone. You can, however, exercise a certain amount of choice when it comes to the decisions you make within your own home. Below are some practical suggestions as to how you can set about creating an energy-balancing, sensually pleasing atmosphere at home. To simplify matters, we will be looking at each of the five senses in turn.

Light and Colour

Most us will already be aware that the colours we are exposed to every day can affect our mood. Some shades, sometimes without your being conscious of it, can make you feel positive and uplifted, while others can make you feel lacklustre and flat. And the presence or absence of light can do much the same. Being deprived of regular sunlight can make you feel depressed and unmotivated. When this becomes clinical depression, it is known as seasonal affective disorder (SAD). Bearing this is in mind, the following tips can help you to feel positive and energized:

- Consciously make use of lighting effects to create a relaxing or stimulating mood, depending on what feels appropriate. If natural light is at a premium, replace conventional light bulbs with those that mimic the effect of daylight.

- If you feel sluggish in the morning and it's an ongoing struggle to haul yourself out of bed, use an alarm clock that mimics the effect of dawning light, rather than relying on the sensory shock of a shrill buzz or ringing.

- If SAD is a diagnosed condition that affects you every winter, sabotaging your energy levels and overall vitality, invest in a full-spectrum lightbox to keep the blues at bay.

- Use colour deliberately to lift mood and create a sense of emotional balance. The following colour choices can be applied to home furnishings, the shades you use for

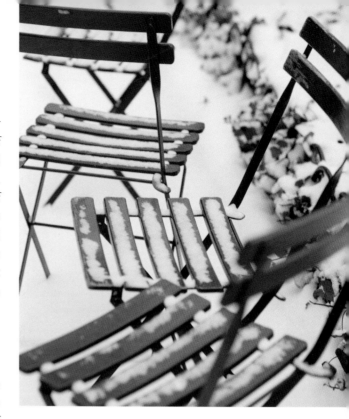

ABOVE **WINTER CAN BE A STRESSFUL SEASON FOR THOSE WHO SUFFER FROM SEASONAL AFFECTIVE DISORDER (SAD).**

decorating your walls and even the clothes that you wear. Below is a brief rundown of some of the qualities that different colours can have:

- **RED** is thought to be stimulating, revitalizing and passionate. As a result, it's a shade that's best not overdone, otherwise it can produce an overstimulating, tiring effect. Small amounts in the bedroom, on the other hand, may be just what's needed as a passion boost.
- **ORANGE** appears to encourage confidence, vitality and outgoing, sociable feelings.
- **YELLOW** is felt to have uplifting, revitalizing effects.
- **GREEN** is regarded as a powerful mood balancer, stimulating feelings of harmony and calm.
- **BLUE** appears to be one of the most relaxation-inducing hues, without creating a soporific effect.
- **INDIGO** or **DARK BLUE** isn't a shade that you are likely to use in large quantities because it's so intense. Judicious use of small amounts of this colour (perhaps a few cushions or a throw), however, is thought to work well in a bedroom or any other place where you want a strongly relaxing, meditative effect.

Sound

So many of us are assaulted on a regular basis by a range of undesirable, disruptive noise that we have to filter it out unconsciously, or we simply wouldn't be able to cope. Common sources of unwelcome noise include burglar and car alarms, telephones, voices raised in argument, overhead flight paths and road repairs. Exposure to unwelcome, disruptive sounds can leave your nerves feeling jangled and on edge without your even realizing it, which, in turn, can leave you feeling drained and stressed. You can't switch off much of this surrounding noise, so you do need to make sure that you enjoy the benefits of exposure to mood-balancing sound whenever you can as a positive compensation.

- Music has potent mood-changing or mood-enhancing qualities that you can tap into whenever you need to. If you're feeling low, listening to your favourite upbeat CD can rapidly make you feel more positive. There may be other times when all you want is to listen to something soothing and classical, or tear-jerking and sentimental. Don't be afraid to expand your current listening habits, as it's very easy to become stuck in a music rut. Finding a new style of music or a fresh new artist can bring an enormous amount of sensual pleasure.

- Don't feel that New Age or classical music is the only companion to inducing a state of emotional harmony and balance. Sometimes total quiet is just what's needed.

- Wind chimes can create a soft, magical, ethereal effect for very little outlay and expense. They don't have to be terribly solemn either. Chimes come in a variety of styles and sizes that can range from intensely tasteful, minimalist shapes to wacky, cat-shaped chimes.

- The sound of water can be either soothing or energizing, depending on your mood at the time. Water features can be used in your garden, on a patio or terrace, or inside your home to create a pleasing visual and auditory effect. Don't forget to take care with regard to the safety of children and small animals if you do choose to have an ambitious water feature indoors.

BELOW **THE GENTLE SOUND OF SPLASHING WATER CAN HAVE A WONDERFULLY SOOTHING EFFECT ON FRAYED NERVES.**

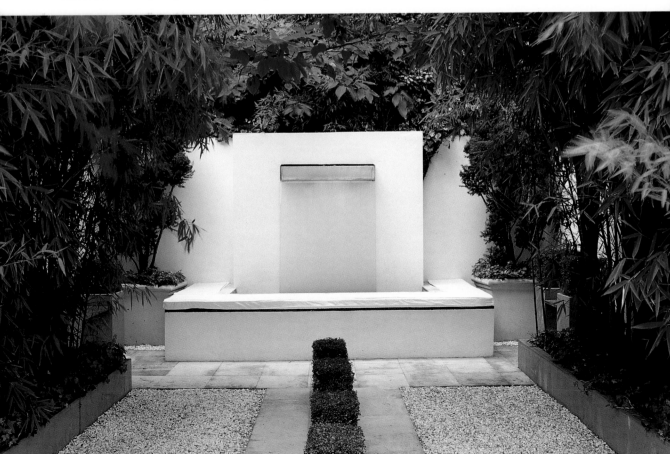

Smell

Perfumes and scents are known to have a powerful effect on our mood and emotions. They are also very evocative. An unexpected whiff of a specific aroma can suddenly conjure up a moment from the past very vividly. Particular smells can make us feel wistful, euphoric, homesick, joyful or bereft depending on their associations for us as individuals. One of the most effective ways of harnessing the powerful mood-influencing impact of scent is to use essential oils imaginatively. Astonishingly concentrated in nature, just a few drops of an essential oil can be burnt in a custom-made essential-oil vaporizer to deliver a sensory pick-me-up whenever you feel low. If you want a simpler approach, sprinkle a few drops onto a tissue or handkerchief, and inhale whenever you feel in need of an energy boost.

- **CITRUS-BASED OILS** such as grapefruit, lemon and orange are refreshing, uplifting and stress-busting.

- **ROSEMARY** is reputedly excellent for clearing the head when you are feeling dull and tired. It's also thought to have aphrodisiac properties.

- **PEPPERMINT** is also well known for its refreshing, stimulating effect. It can be especially helpful if you have a problem waking up in the morning.

- **PETITGRAIN** has a refreshing aroma that's thought to ease stress-related symptoms such as insomnia, nervous exhaustion and fatigue.

- **LAVENDER** has uplifting, calming and refreshing properties.

- **CLARY SAGE** has a reputation as a mood-balancing aroma that can be reviving or relaxing. It's also thought to help stimulate libido.

- **GERANIUM** has a piercing, sweet, slightly minty perfume. It is refreshing and uplifting when you're jaded and low.

RIGHT VAPORIZERS CAN BE USED TO RELEASE THE SCENT OF DIFFERENT ESSENTIAL OILS DEPENDING ON YOUR MOOD.

Homemade Room Spray

A natural, refreshing room spray can be made by adding a sparing amount of essential oil to a small plastic or glass plant mister. Approximately 18 drops of essential oil should be added to about ½ cup (125 ml/4 fl oz) of tap water. This spray can then be used whenever a room seems to smell less than inviting – for instance, after a party when the aroma of stale cigarette smoke is lingering or if your home has been shut up all day. Try one or both of the following combinations:

- Three drops of geranium, three drops of petitgrain, and five drops each of lemon and bergamot

- Six drops of lavender, four drops of peppermint and five drops of clary sage

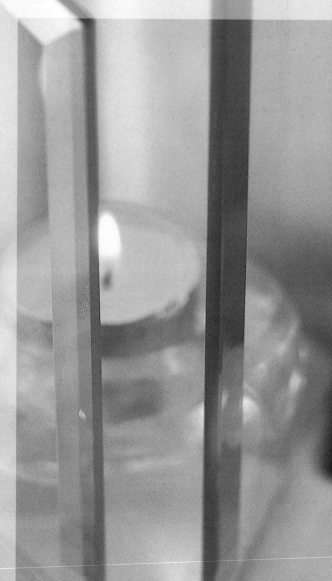

Touch

Desired touch is one of the most sensual pleasures we can ever know. We can experience a deep state of arousal, comfort and closeness as a result of physical contact from someone whom we love and trust. Sadly, the pleasure of touch can be one of the most neglected whenever you feel stressed, tired or under pressure. If matters get out of hand, you can arrive at a point where even responding to another's touch can begin to feel like just another demand. As a result, you may feel lonely, guilty, cut off and generally out of synch with those around you.

The good news is that the situation is reversible; all it takes is some conscious effort to get your relationship back on track again. Once you make the time to do this, you're likely to find that you feel energized and liberated, as you will be able to get back in touch with your emotions and those of your partner once again. All it requires is the willingness to put aside some time and a little ingenuity.

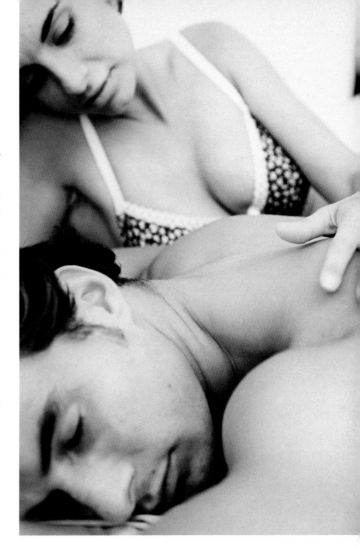

- It's easy to get into the habit of only touching or looking at our partner when we make love, with the result that we lose a basic sense of physical closeness. If you watch how spontaneously children express themselves through touch and receive affection so openly, it can really come home to you that you are missing out hugely if you've lost the ability to touch. Holding hands, hugging or putting a comforting arm around a shoulder can communicate so much more than a host of words.

- Making time for each other is a must if loving, sensual communication is to take place. How many of us find through pressure of time that we only half listen to what our partner is saying because we're trying to get the children ready for school, thinking ahead to that difficult presentation we're about to give or zoning out in front of the television? If we're honest, we've all been there. This needn't be a major problem unless not listening properly becomes a frequent habit. On the other hand, feeling that you're not being listened to on a daily basis can be one of the things that undermines a relationship at its core. If you have any doubts about this, just watch how lovers behave at the outset of an intense relationship. They don't just touch, but make frequent eye contact and really pay attention to what their partner is saying. Listening and being heard are common casualties of a long-term relationship if we aren't careful, and they need to be woven back into your love life if you are to experience the sensual pleasure of truly communicating.

- Resist the habit of making love at the end of the day purely from habit. While this may suit some of us, there is a good chance that by this point of your day you're both more interested in falling asleep than enjoying a passionate encounter. Be imaginative and choose a time of day that suits both partners so that energy levels are going to be high. You don't have to be Olympic or tantric marathon lovers, but you do need to have enough vitality to ensure that you don't merely go through the motions.

ABOVE **TOUCH IS THE MOST IMMEDIATE AND INTIMATE FORM OF COMMUNICATION.**

- Sensual massage can be a powerful, immediate way of communicating with your partner. Set aside plenty of time so that there's no sense of being rushed or forced, and make sure that the room is comfortably warm. Lighting should be soft and imaginative: lighting scented candles can be an excellent way of creating a sensually pleasing effect. Don't worry about not being an expert in massage: it's much more important to be aware of how your partner is responding than to be preoccupied with whether you're getting the strokes just right. Use a massage oil to help the gliding movements of your hands smoothly and evenly over the body. Ready-made blends are easily available, or you can make your own by adding six drops of ylang ylang or sandalwood essential oil to four teaspoons of carrier oil. Always warm the oil in your hands before you begin to apply it so that you avoid dripping cold oil onto your partner's body. This can have a slightly jarring rather than an erotic effect. The pressure and pattern of strokes are up to you and your partner, but common massage techniques include gentle circling, stroking, kneading and cupping movements.

- Encourage sensual awareness by noticing everyday sensations that are often taken for granted. These could be something as simple as the pleasure of slipping into fresh, fragrant bedsheets or savouring the feel of a soft, slinky fabric against your skin.

- It can be immensely relaxing to have a full-body massage from a trained therapist every once in a while to help keep stress levels in balance and let go of tense, tight muscles. This can be especially important if you live alone and are liable to feel cut off and lonely. If you don't have enough time or cash for a full-body treatment, make a point of having a neck, shoulder and back massage instead.

Taste

The energy-boosting or vitality-draining properties of food and drink have already been dealt with in chapter 3 (see pages 54–73). Nevertheless, there are some additional sensible tips in relation to our eating habits that it is important to bear in mind as part of any energizing plan, particular when it comes to savouring the taste and texture of food.

- It may seem to be stating the obvious, but it's very important to take time to savour all the tastes and flavours of any meal that you're eating. Gulping down a sandwich on the run or collapsing in front of the television with a ready-made meal and a can of cola are guaranteed to do very little for you in the energy-boosting stakes. Habits such as these are more likely to land you with indigestion and heartburn. After all, if you don't chew food thoroughly because you're concentrating on something else, you're also likely to find that you eat more than you actually need because you're distracted. On the other hand, if you take the time to sit down to a meal and pay attention to the various tastes and textures, you are likely to enjoy the experience much more, while also allowing your digestive system to work as it should and avoiding overeating by being alert to the first sensation of fullness.

- Take time to appreciate the visual appearance of food and its tantalizing aromas as it is being prepared. Apart from the sensual pleasure that this brings, it also benefits the digestive system. The digestion process is activated by the secretion of enzymes as your mouth waters in preparation for eating. As a result, taking pleasure in the smell and appearance of food readies your digestive system even before you've put a morsel of food into your mouth.

- Food can be an emotional minefield, with much of the pleasure of eating being tainted by feelings of guilt or self-indulgence. This can especially be the case if you see food as fattening and dangerous. An unhealthy concern with weight loss at the expense of a healthy pleasure in eating can lead to an unbalanced relationship with food. Putting the principles of healthy eating into practice (i.e. concentrating on high-fibre, complex carbohydrates, fresh, raw fruit and vegetables, small amounts of protein, and lots of filtered water) will often stabilize your weight naturally and ensure that you enjoy sustained levels of energy. At all costs avoid yo-yo or fad patterns of dieting. These destroy the natural pleasure you deserve to take in eating, while also making it more likely that you'll gain weight in the long run.

RIGHT **FOOD CAN BE A DEEPLY SENSUOUS PLEASURE IF YOU ALLOW YOURSELF ENOUGH TIME TO ENJOY IT.**

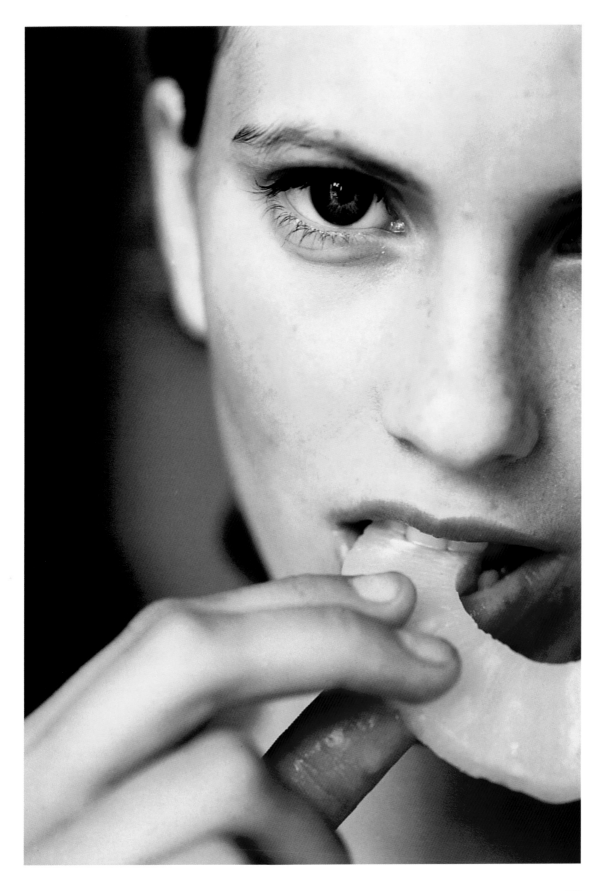

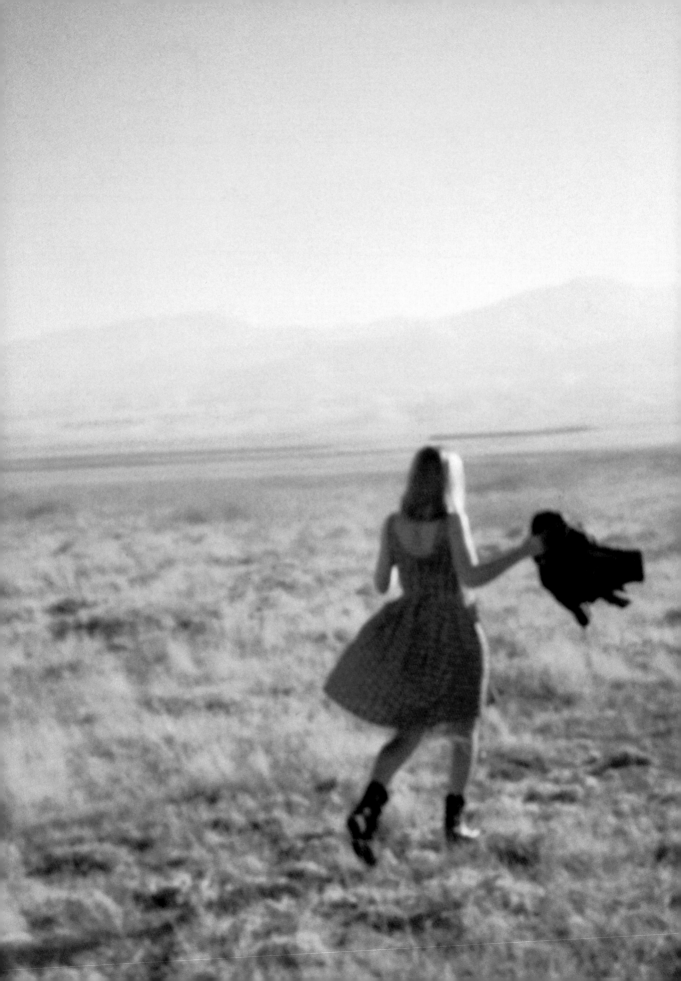

Energy traps

There are definite pitfalls that you need to avoid when you are under pressure. The following are some practical suggestions designed for use whenever you are feeling a bit sluggish and need to shake things up.

Clutter clearing

Nothing is quite so energy-draining as feeling that you are surrounded by a variety of jobs that you've been putting off for ages. Piles of papers yet to be dealt with, heaps of clothes that haven't been worn for ages but still haven't been sorted out, assorted clutter on the floor – all can contribute to the feeling that you are not in control. Taking a proactive stance with regard to tasks that have been bothering you for too long can inject you with a boost of energy and vitality. You may find that you need to do them all in one fell swoop – if you respond well to this approach, it may be that you usually need the stimulation of a tight deadline to get you moving. You may need to do small amounts steadily and slowly. Whatever your method, ensure that you bag everything to be thrown out and get rid of it straight away. If you don't, you'll trade heaps of junk for large black, plastic bags full of junk. From a feng shui perspective, ridding yourself of unwanted items allows energy to flow so that you are free to move in fresh directions.

Electric gadgets

If tiredness is a constant problem on waking, it's worth assessing how many electrical appliances you have in your bedroom. It may be that you have unwittingly overloaded your bedroom

with a television, CD player, electric clock, electric blanket and other appliances, disturbing your biomagnetic energy. If this seems to be the case, simply remove any unnecessary electrical objects, or swap them for a nonelectrical variety. For instance, an electric blanket can be traded for an old-fashioned hot-water bottle, while a television set is best enjoyed outside the bedroom. Watching television in bed can lead to tension headaches from poor posture and difficulty in sleeping as a result of too much stimulation late at night.

Achieving optimum balance

When the pressure is on, it is all too easy to forget that you need to be striving for a sense of balance in your life. So, if you're working and/or playing extra hard, you need to make sure that you're making time for yourself to chill out and replenish your basic levels of energy and dynamism. It really doesn't matter how you choose to spend this time: some of us may choose to try some of the specific relaxation techniques outlined in the following chapter, while others will prefer to indulge in something spontaneously that they find has a soothing, replenishing effect. It all depends on individual taste and any of the following could help. Soak in a soothing bath scented with aromatherapy oils, take a long walk in the country or along a beach, go to a movie, enjoy a laugh with friends, or make a point of having regular early nights tucked up in bed with a favourite book. The main aim is to ensure that you have enough replenishing time to recharge those energy batteries, especially at times when you know that you're going to be under more pressure than usual.

Above all, never feel guilty about taking restorative time out for just you. Doing this is not an indulgence, but rather a practical way of ensuring you keep a healthy balance in your life.

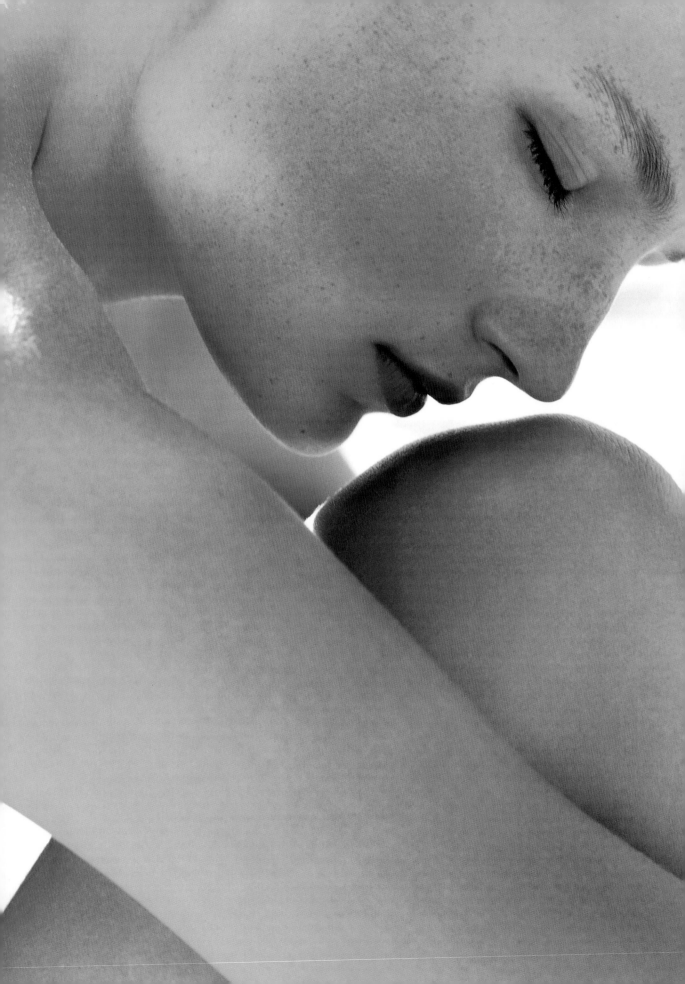

6 Creative spirit

Just as you need to nurture your body by eating well and exercising regularly, if you're to ensure that you enjoy optimum levels of energy and an abundant sense of vitality, you also need to pay attention to balancing your emotions.

Emotions such as anger, anxiety and sadness can have a powerfully draining effect on your energy levels without you even noticing, leaving you feeling exhausted and on an emotional short fuse most of the time. If you have effectively suppressed these feelings, you will typically find yourself inexplicably overreacting to the smallest of triggers – which in itself uses up a substantial reserves of energy, adding to your feeling drained and exhausted.

If this scenario sounds all too familiar, don't despair. There are simple techniques at your disposal that can support you in effectively diffusing some of the most common mental and emotional energy drainers such as anxiety, depression, irritability or guilt. This chapter explores some very practical, straightforward techniques that can help you to begin your process of liberation from this sort of emotional straitjacket. There is additional advice in the following chapter (see pages 110–23) on alternative medical approaches that can provide a gentle form of extra support when you need it.

LEFT **INNER STRENGTH IS NEVER FAR AWAY, YOU JUST NEED TO KNOW HOW TO ACCESS IT.**

BANISHING THE FOUR ANTI-ENERGY DEMONS

Depression

Depressive feelings are among the most powerful destructive influences in our lives, creating symptoms of exhaustion, negativity, lack of motivation and downright despair. The strength and duration of these feelings can vary enormously, depending on whether you are suffering from clinical depression or a short-lived bout of the 'blues'. The advice that's offered below is primarily aimed at those who fall into the second category, but if you are a long-term sufferer of depression you may still gain some helpful insights. Clinical depression, however, is a chronic illness that requires professional support and attention – either through medication or 'talking' therapies, or a combination of both. Any self-help measures should be viewed as additional rather than alternative help.

- **If a bout of the 'blues' has descended and your natural response is to cut yourself off from those that you care for most, think again. Being alone can sometimes be helpful; however, when you're feeling depressed, having no one around can increase your feelings of isolation. Instead, be honest about how you're feeling with a good, sympathetic listener. Voicing your feelings in this way can often help you to see your situation in a more balanced light.**

- Having a good laugh or a cry on a sympathetic shoulder can also help at times. Often when depressive feelings descend, you judge yourself very harshly and think that others don't need to be burdened with your feelings. When you have genuinely good, sympathetic friends, nothing could be further from the truth, as they are likely to react positively to a cry for help or emotional support.

- Sleep patterns can be disturbed when you're feeling down. You can either sleep for too long and feel lethargic and sluggish as a result, or you may wake too early feeling unrefreshed and jittery. If either of these tendencies develops, see the advice given in the section on insomnia on page 114 to try to improve the depth and pattern of sleep. This is crucial to protect your basic energy levels.

- When you feel low, always eat well and regularly. Difficult as it may be to muster up the motivation, it really is worth the effort. Blood sugar levels play an important role in contributing to mood swings. Although not the root cause of feeling low, if your blood sugar levels are erratic, this can lead to additional symptoms of jitteriness, irritability, anxiety, poor concentration and low mental and emotional energy. This certainly won't help the situation if you're already feeling mentally and emotionally vulnerable and fragile. For practical, easy-to-apply advice on balancing blood sugar levels, see chapter 3 (pages 54–73).

- Aerobic exercise is an important tool in helping you to fight the blues. It needn't involve anything more ambitious than taking a brisk walk each day lasting roughly 30 to 45 minutes. If cycling or running suits you better, these are also fine. What is crucial is that it is aerobic exercise. Using the large muscles in your arms and legs while engaging in rhythmic, continuous activity conditions your heart, lungs and circulatory and lymphatic systems, while also boosting the body's secretion of feel-good endorphins.

- If you're low and 'blue' because you're feeling generally negative, it can be almost second nature to blame yourself for how you feel. This only leads to additional feelings of guilt or blame. The whole point of depressive feelings is that they can descend independently of our conscious control. As a result, one of the worst things to say to someone who's struggling with depressive feelings is

to 'pull themselves together'. When you feel low, try to see yourself as a basically good person trying the best they can to cope with negative feelings. Cut yourself some emotional slack. Treat yourself the way you'd treat a close friend or family member if they felt the same way. This isn't self-indulgence, but an intrinsic part of a survival strategy.

- Burn aromatherapy oils in a custom-made vaporizer to help balance mood and lift a sense of feeling emotionally flat. Oils to choose from include any of the following: camomile, clary sage, ylang ylang, lavender and marjoram.

- Herbal support is available in the form of St John's Wort for mild bouts of feeling 'blue'. If you are taking prescription drugs, it's essential that you seek the advice of your doctor or a pharmacist before starting treatment with St John's Wort. It can render some conventional drugs less effective, including conventional antidepressants, epilepsy drugs, medication for heart disorders, some asthma drugs, HIV treatment, conventional migraine medications, and anti-clotting or anti-rejection medication.

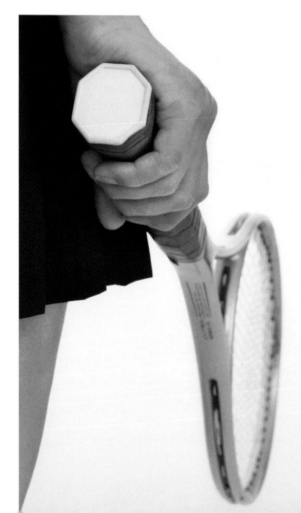

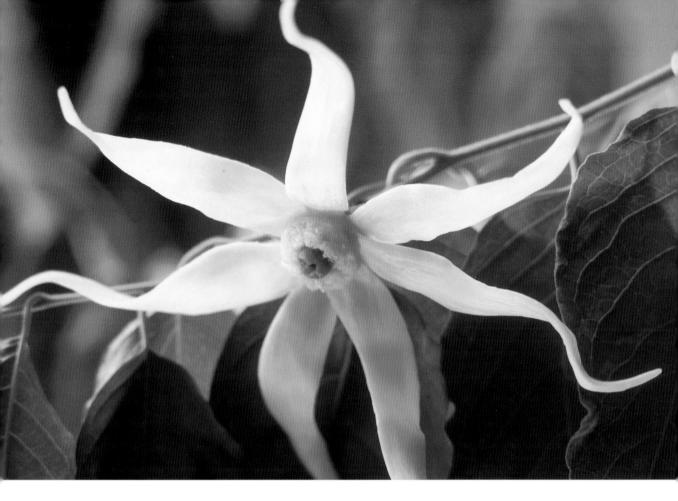

Anxiety

Your body uses up a huge amount of nervous energy if you suffer from frequent problems with anxiety. This is partly due to a stress mechanism called the 'fight-or-flight' response, which is triggered whenever we feel under threat. What this means is that, when you're under strain, your body automatically reacts by preparing to engage in physical combat or sprint away from the source of danger. While this can be a very effective way of dealing with a problem if either of these courses of action is appropriate, most of the stresses you're likely to find yourself confronted with on a regular basis – arguments with your partner or confronting an unusually large bill, for instance – can't be dealt with in this way.

LEFT **REGULAR EXERCISE CAN PLAY A VITAL PART IN DEALING WITH A MILD TO MODERATE BOUT OF DEPRESSION.**
ABOVE **ALWAYS USE MOOD-BALANCING ESSENTIAL OILS SPARINGLY AS THEY ARE HIGHLY CONCENTRATED.**

As a result, regular tripping of the fight-or-flight response is going to make you feel edgy, jittery and tense owing to the stress hormones flooding your body that are not being burned off by physical activity. This leads to constantly tight, aching muscles, recurrent headaches, reduced appetite, stomach cramps, poor sleep pattern, palpitations and possibly panic attacks if the process is allowed to continue for too long. As you can imagine, all of these critically diminish your reserves.

The advice given below is invaluable if you feel pretty calm on a day-to-day basis, but find that, if the pressure heats up, you start to feel uncomfortably on edge. If you've reached the stage of occasional panic attacks, there is specific advice coping with these in the next chapter (see page 113).

Counselling can also play an important part in alleviating anxiety that has descended after you have been through a period of excessive stress or bereavement. Most crucially of all, discovering that you are not alone and that many other people have suffered similar feelings can be a huge relief.

Breathing through anxiety

Calming breathing techniques can be powerful allies, enabling you to switch on the relaxation response when you're beginning to feel uptight. If you feel stressed and under pressure, you will tend to breathe rapidly and in a shallow fashion from your upper chest. You may also clench your jaw, while also holding your shoulders rigidly as an unconscious form of 'body armouring'. This has the combined effect of making you feel even more jittery and on edge, as the proportion between oxygen and carbon dioxide in your bloodstream becomes unbalanced.

The good news is that you can turn the situation around, leading you quickly to feel calmer, relaxed and more in control. All this takes is a little concentration and conscious effort to begin breathing slowly and steadily, using your full lung capacity.

You can learn how to do this by placing a hand on your belly roughly just above your navel area. As you breathe in, consciously relaxing the chest and filling your lungs from the base to the top, you should sense your upper chest rising until it reaches the point where your hand rises slightly upwards and outwards. This is an indication that your lungs are being used to maximum capacity. Wait a second before releasing a full breath, with the hand moving back to its original position as your lungs empty themselves fully.

With practice, this form of slow, complete breathing should no longer feel forced, but instead flow in a steady, rhythmical way, rather like a wave that naturally flows upon the shore then back to the sea in a seemingly effortless motion. Never strain the process, but take enough time to allow it to feel natural, and always stop and breathe normally for a little while if you start to feel light-headed or dizzy.

Tips for Coping with Anxiety

- Some foods and drinks have a reputation for aggravating symptoms of anxiety. It is best to avoid these entirely or at least cut down on them drastically at times of high pressure. The usual suspects include the following: coffee, fizzy and caffeinated drinks, chocolate, tea, alcohol and sugar-rich items such as confectionery, cakes, biscuits (cookies) and convenience foods.

- Simple as it sounds, one of the most effective ways of banishing nagging, minor worries is to envision how much of a problem that particular issue is going to pose in two, five or ten years time. The chances are that this technique will help you to put problems that have moved out of perspective into a more realistic frame.

- Sometimes specific situations or particular phobias can trigger anxiety, and this can have a limiting effect on your whole life. For instance, a terror of giving public presentations can hold someone back from a deserved promotion at work, or a fear of flying can make it difficult

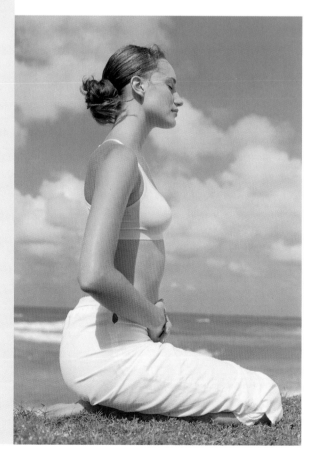

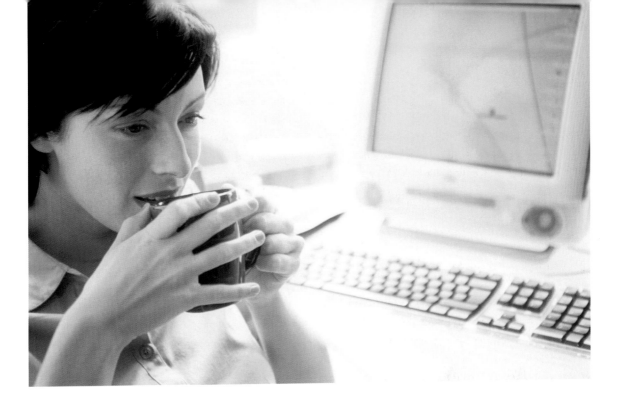

ABOVE **THOSE EXTRA CUPS OF COFFEE CAN QUICKLY GROW TO A FULL-SCALE PROBLEM. TRY SOOTHING DRINKS INSTEAD.** LEFT **CONTROLLED BREATHING TECHNIQUES CAN BE A HUGE SUPPORT IN BANISHING FEELINGS OF ANXIETY AND PANIC.**

to travel to certain destinations on holiday. If this is true in your case, it can be very helpful to consult a psychologist. Techniques used by behavioural psychologists can be very useful in teaching you ways of slowly confronting the source of your anxiety and fear, so that you can conquer it in time. This approach can give you a huge sense of liberation when you discover that the object or situation that you've been so terror-stricken about is in fact not so dreadful after all, and that you possess the courage to cope with it.

- When you do feel anxious and jittery, you can be strongly tempted to start thinking in terms of 'catastrophe.' In other words, you begin to imagine the problems you're feeling anxious about setting off a series of disastrous events, resulting in a catastrophe further down the line. It's amazing how fertile our imaginations can be when supplying us with the details of such a major disaster. This may well be a common response, but it is unfortunately resoundingly unhelpful when a problem needs to be solved. If you do find yourself starting to think in these terms, you aren't going to feel empowered to make any

rational decisions about how to deal with whatever it is that's bothering you. In fact, quite the reverse is true, as spending emotional energy on fretting about something that isn't likely to happen will only make you feel more upset and exhausted than you need to. You need to stop this doomsaying in its tracks. First, identify that it is happening, as you can't solve a problem unless you acknowledge that it's there in the first place. Whenever the first signs appear, take mental and emotional action, putting a halt to the process. This will probably feel difficult and unnatural at first, but the rewards that follow are well worth the effort.

- Practising being in the present moment can help you enormously if you have a tendency to free-floating anxiety that attaches itself to any worry that is passing by at the time. Focusing your attention on what is happening right now will mean that you are going to experience a great deal more pleasure in the present. It also prevents you from projecting your thoughts forward in a negative way. This is very important, as there's every chance that solutions will present themselves when the event actually arrives that your past experience hasn't allowed for. It also helps to bear in mind that taking action to solve a problem when you're actually confronted with the reality of it is much less stressful than imagining problems that you can't take any positive action to solve.

103

Anger

We seem to be living in an increasingly angry society. Escalating problems with road rage, random acts of violence and the breakdown of relationships all seem to indicate that unresolved anger is contributing to a sense of general emotional dislocation. Not that appropriately expressed anger, in itself, need be negative. In fact, expressing justified unhappiness and anger in a controlled and assertive way can be much healthier than suppressing these powerful emotions, as they're likely to fester and seethe under the surface.

If this happens, you are likely to experience the dual problems of feeling emotionally drained and uneasy much of the time, without understanding why. These buried feelings can act like a time bomb. All it takes is an unsuspecting person who unwittingly puts their foot in it and ends up on the receiving end of a tirade that seems totally unjustified or out of proportion.

The following are helpful practical tools that you can use to manage anger in the future. Once you're liberated from an emotional 'short-fuse' reaction, you will be amazed how much more emotional resilience and energy you have at your disposal. As a bonus, you're almost certainly going to find the world a much more relaxing and inviting place.

• Whenever you feel irritated or downright angry about something, do a quick reality check to assess whether your reaction is justified. Take a few relaxing breaths (see page 102) to clear your head before assessing the situation. If on quick but considered reflection it really does seem justified to express your anger, do it in an assertive but not abusive way at the time of the incident. Otherwise there is a danger that these feelings will fester below the surface to explode at a later date. On the other hand, if it looks as if you are losing your sense of perspective, simply take a few more calming breaths before mentally moving on.

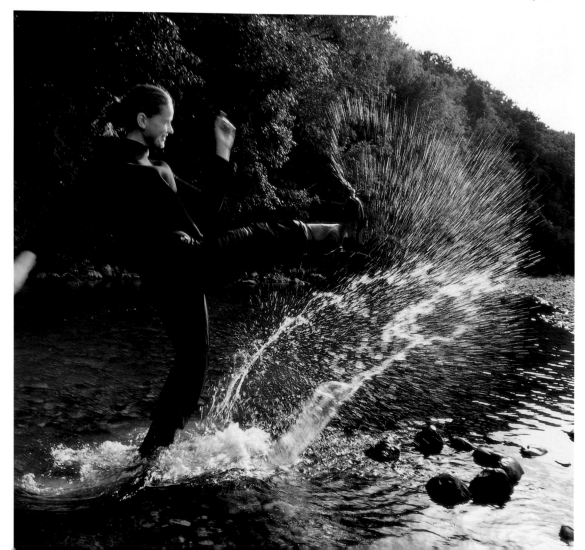

- Depression can descend if you turn unresolved anger inwards for too long. This can have the undesirable effect of damaging your self-esteem and personal power, with the result that you feel extremely negative about yourself and your capabilities. If you do feel you're being drained of emotional and physical energy as a result of a negative self-image, consider exploring this with the support of a trained counsellor, psychotherapist or homeopath.

- Certain foods and drinks can contribute to feeling on a 'short fuse'. You would do well to steer clear of them when you feel angry and uptight. See the list under in the anxiety section on page 102 for a guide to foods and drinks to avoid. Unstable blood sugar levels can also make you feel irritable and snappy, so it's worth taking a look at the Zappers section in chapter 3 (pages 57–60).

- If you're alone and want to let off steam safely, try punching a cushion, singing or doing a vigorous exercise workout such as Tae-Bo.

Guilt

An inappropriate sense of guilt can be one of the most draining emotions you experience. Carrying around unresolved guilt with you on a day-to-day basis can poison the present, leaving you unable to relax and take pleasure in the moment. Guilty feelings can be associated with displaced anxiety. For instance, you may be unable to enjoy a carefree day out because you feel a lurking sense of worry that you didn't check that all the electrical appliances at home were switched off. As a result, if something goes wrong, you feel that it is your fault.

Guilt felt in appropriate situations can prevent us from becoming amoral, selfish or exploiting others. But many of us are hampered by unnecessary feelings of remorse that hold us back from leading a creative, balanced life. If this is due to emotional baggage that you've been carrying with you from childhood, it can be extremely liberating to try to identify when these negative patterns were laid

LEFT SOMETIMES WE JUST NEED TO LET OFF SOME STEAM BY DOING SOMETHING EXHILARATING.

down. Were you made to feel special, loved and secure as a child, or were you given subtle signals that love and affection were conditional? Or have you been left with lingering feelings that you were criticized, undervalued or overlooked?

Sadly, if you have carried these impressions around with you from an early age, there's a strong chance that you will always feel under pressure to reach increasingly difficult or unachievable goals in order to win the love, attention and respect of those you care for most. The result of this emotional programming is almost certainly going to be a growing sense of insecurity, failure, guilt and inadequacy as you fall short of the standards you set yourself. Escaping from this cycle entails recognizing that this is the case. Once you identify the problem, you will be empowered to take steps to resolve it.

- The first stage in changing unmerited patterns of guilt involves standing back whenever you feel familiar feelings of uneasiness descending. Assess how realistic the guilty response actually is in proportion to the situation. You are likely to feel either that you've done the best job that you could in the circumstances or that you may perhaps have made some mistakes, but they aren't life-shattering. If the latter seems to be true, you can use this insight to your advantage. Learn from the experience, so that you're better placed to deal with something similar in the future.

- If persistent feelings of guilt revolve around a particular person or situation, evaluate as objectively as you can how realistic your responses are. On reflection, you may feel that you can do more to help the situation along by taking a positive, proactive approach. Or you may come to the conclusion that you really have done as much positive work as possible under the circumstances, but that you're not receiving the basic support you need in order to resolve the situation successfully. If this appears to be the case, consciously let go of the situation and move on.

- Above all, if your self-esteem is low, don't fall into the common trap of feeling guilty when a compliment is paid to you. Strive to accept it at face value and gain pleasure from it, rather than looking for any hidden motives. You really should give yourself permission to be happy.

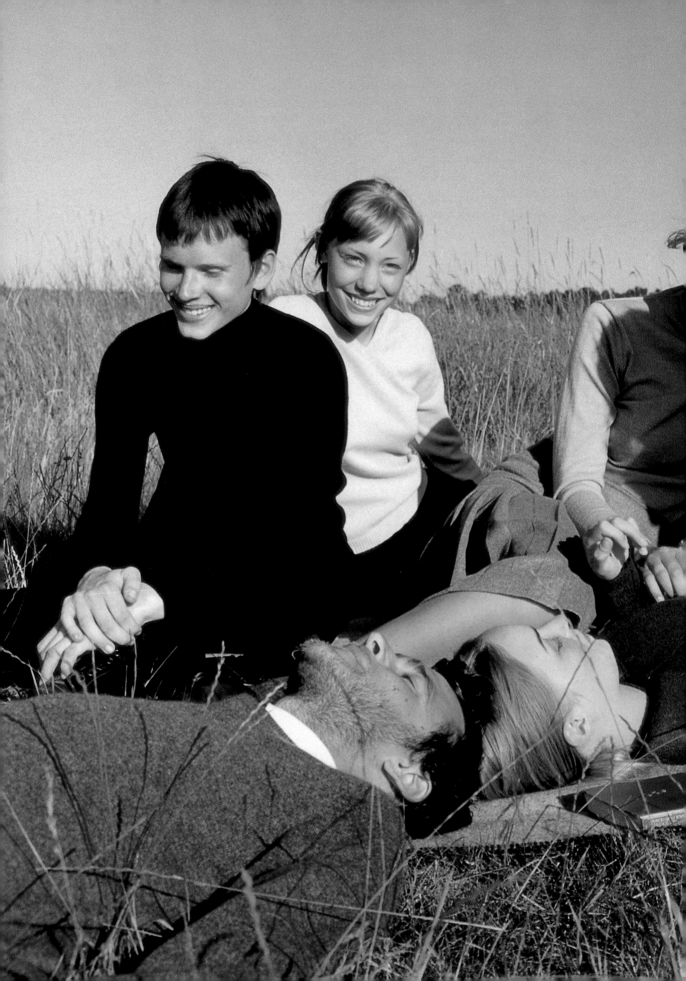

Ten simple steps to positive thinking

If you instinctively bring a negative perspective to your day-to-day life, you're likely to be squandering a great deal of mental energy worrying about a negative outcome in advance of any event. By contrast, if you consciously bring an open, realistically positive perspective to a situation, you can do a significant amount to influence a positive outcome. This inevitably boosts your sense of overall confidence and optimism, both of which are fundamentally energizing feelings.

The next time a challenging situation presents itself, stop for a moment and observe your initial reaction to it. If, after a while, you notice that your first reaction is repeatedly a mainly pessimistic one, consciously consider an alternative, more upbeat perspective. This may feel very unnatural and demanding at first, but the opening up of positive possibilities as a result will be well worth the effort.

1   A positive perspective can only emerge when you take a balanced view of any situation, rather than automatically taking a downbeat approach to problem solving.

2   Try to be as flexible and adaptable as possible when considering potential solutions to problems, rather than feeling completely devastated if plan A doesn't work. Always consider what your safety-net solution is going to be (plan B). If this doesn't materialize, bring plans C and D into play.

3   What is your response to the idea of change most likely to be? Always be aware that change in itself is often neutral: it's the perspective you bring to it that determines whether you see it as a chance for new opportunities or as a threat. If you learn to embrace inevitable change, you have a far greater chance of turning it into an enriching experience.

4   Whenever a stressful or challenging event is approaching, instead of fretting about it try visualizing yourself accomplishing the task calmly, positively and successfully.

5   If previous experiences of failure or disappointment have put you off attempting something similar, stop for a moment to consider a fresh way of reacting. Instead of avoiding the situation, learn from the previous problems. Use this important information to tackle a similar experience from a position of increased power.

6   Using positive, concrete ways of expressing yourself can change the way in which you see an issue and the way in which others see you approaching it. For example, if you're asked to do something, it is much more assertive to say 'Yes, I will' or 'No, I'm really sorry, but I can't', rather than 'Maybe, but I'm really not sure' or 'I'll try', knowing full well that it's not going to happen.

7   If you're feeling harassed because your stress levels are rising sharply, it helps enormously to take a moment to yourself, rather than just letting the accumulating pressure get to you. You may need no more than five minutes of anxiety-reducing breathing techniques or a quick break by yourself with a cup of stress-reducing herbal tea. The most important thing is to allow yourself to enjoy the interval that you need so that you come away from it refreshed and more in command.

8   If something positive happens, don't simply move on to the next task without pause. Take a little time to bask in the moment. Most important of all, don't be afraid to congratulate yourself on what you've achieved, big or small.

9   Deliberately spend time in the company of people who make you feel uplifted and positive. This isn't an indulgence, but an important way of boosting your emotional batteries.

10 Don't automatically take the pessimistic view. Remember to consider that almost any situation can be seen from a 'glass half empty' or a 'glass half full' perspective. In other words, even a seemingly disappointing or challenging situation can bring unexpected benefits and insights if you look hard and carefully enough for them.

BOOSTING MENTAL ENERGY

The remarkable benefits that come from regularly practising meditation and relaxation techniques are now well known. The conscious use of regular, guided relaxation has been credited with a reduced tendency to suffer from common stress-related problems such high blood pressure, palpitations, digestive troubles and poor sleep patterns. In addition, there are more general bonuses that are attributed to the regular use of relaxation techniques. These include enhanced mental clarity, greater emotional balance, improved concentration and increased mental productivity and creativity. If you make time for relaxation each day, you will be going a long way towards boosting your mental and emotional energy reserves.

Follow your instincts when choosing how to relax. Some of us may find we do very well with one of the guided relaxation CDs available on the market, while others may prefer to record their own instructions. Whatever path you choose, make sure that the exercise you are listening to enables you to relax and unwind, rather than make you grit your teeth in irritation at the speaker's voice or words.

The following is a simple guided relaxation exercise that you may like to try if you're a newcomer to relaxation. It is ideal for calming your mind and improving mental focus.

- Make sure that the room or space where you carry out this exercise is comfortably warm, well ventilated and as free of distracting noise as possible.

- Lie down on the floor, making sure that your clothes are comfortable, not restrictive and warm enough – your body temperature will drop significantly during relaxation. Ensure that there are no distractions to demand your attention while you are relaxing.

- It can help to adopt the yoga relaxation position called 'the corpse' to ensure that your body makes comfortable contact with the floor. This involves nothing more elaborate than lying on your back with your head and neck as relaxed as possible. Your arms and hands should be straight and slightly extended away from your body, with the backs of your hands resting lightly against the floor and your fingers curled loosely towards your palms. Your legs should also feel loose and fall a small distance away from each other – your feet should be approximately 30cm (12in) apart.

- Once you are comfortable, become aware of your breathing pattern, consciously but gently regulating it in a smooth, steady rhythm.

- Bring your attention first to the muscles of your head and face. Starting at the crown of your head, visualize letting go of any tension you feel in your scalp muscles. Move steadily down your forehead, cheeks, jaw and chin, consciously softening any tight or tense muscles.

- Move down your body slowly and steadily in this way, concentrating particularly on common sites of muscle tension such as the neck, shoulders, and upper and lower back. As you become more familiar with spotting areas of tight muscles, you may be surprised by how much tension you unconsciously hold in areas such as your hands, buttocks, thighs or calf muscles. Once these pockets of energy-draining tightness are identified, let them go mentally and feel them physically relax.

- Once you've worked fully down your body, bring your attention back to your breathing again. You should find that it has naturally slowed itself and instinctively regulated to become a gentle, steady rhythm.

- As you take the next breath, imagine yourself being filled with a golden light that is full of positive energy. Watch it move from the top of your head, down your neck, chest, arms, abdomen and legs, filling your whole body with a sense of balanced energy. As you breathe out, picture any pockets of negative energy leaving your body and being replaced with the golden light.

- In time, you may feel that you want to choose another colour than gold, according to your mood.

- Stay in this calm state for as long as feels comfortable, leaving plenty of time to gradually move out of this deeply

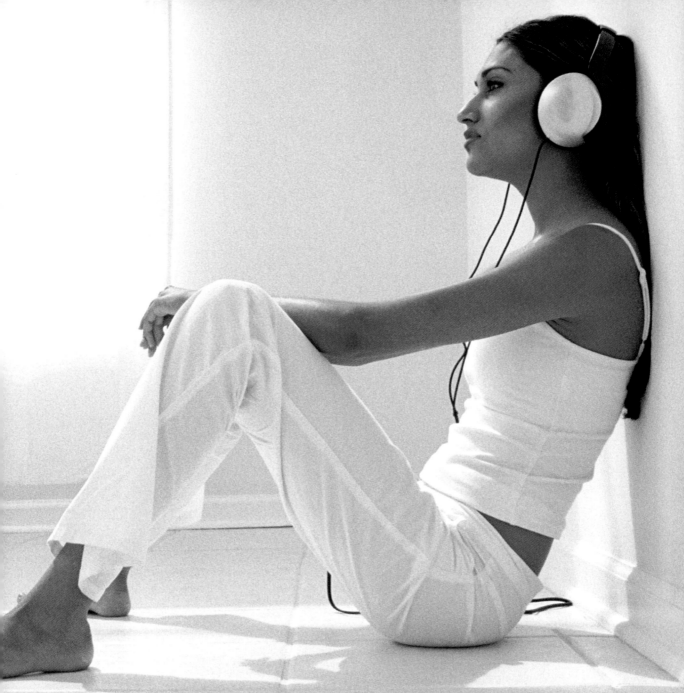

relaxed state. Don't rush. You need to ensure that you reap the full benefits of relaxation.

- When you feel ready, slowly turn your attention to your surroundings. Gently move your head, arms, fingers, legs and feet, making tiny movements at first that gradually build into larger ones. Move in whatever way feels most comfortable to you. This could involve a whole-body stretch or gently cradling your knees into the body.

- Once your eyes are open and you're ready to move, always resist the temptation to move into an upright

ABOVE **LET THE PACE OF RELAXATION COME NATURALLY.**

position abruptly. Instead, take time to roll on one side first, then spend a little time in a sitting position. Finally, curl into an upright position, bringing your head up last.

- To get the most out of conscious relaxation, aim to practise a session every day, even if just a shortened version. For many of us, the best time is just before bed, so that we can prepare for a sound night's sleep. The key thing is to establish it as a regular routine. The benefits are sure to persuade you make it a regular part of your day.

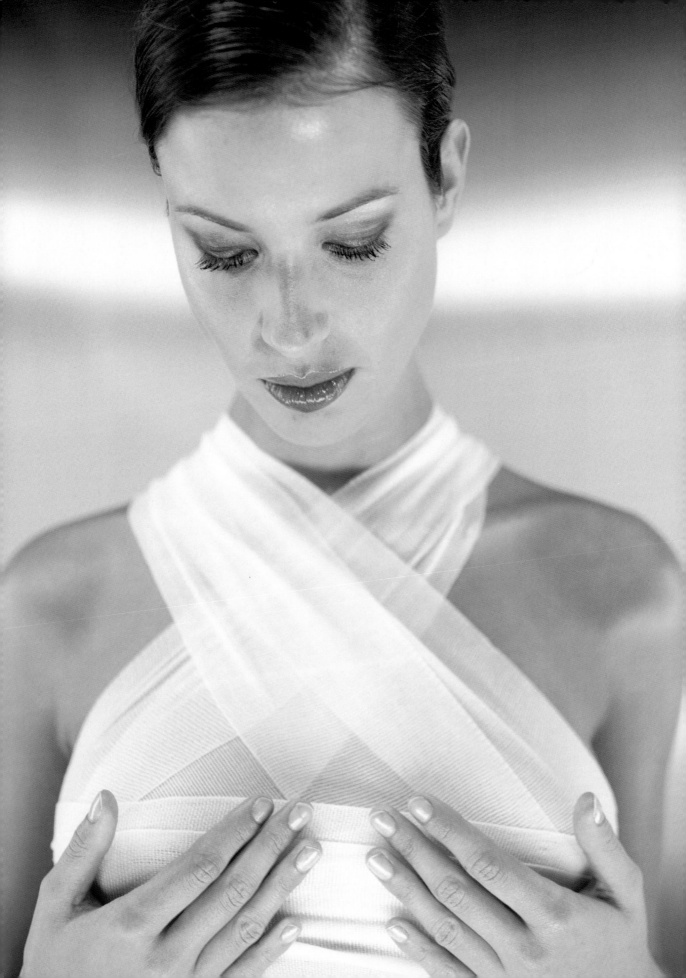

7 Healing power

This chapter is designed to give you some practical, quick-fix hints that you can use if life has temporarily hit the skids. Most of this advice takes the form of alternative and complementary medical self-help; however, in some cases pointers are given when professional help is more appropriate in order to deal successfully with the situation. All of the conditions addressed relate to an imbalance of energy in some way; for convenience sake they have been divided into two main sections. The first of these loosely relates to problems that are often associated with exhaustion that comes from living in the fast lane for too long, while the second group often arise when energy is generally sluggish and easily depleted.

Of course, the following advice is not intended to take the place of conventional medical treatment completely. For instance, if you've been exceptionally tired for an extended period of time for no obvious reason, you must have this checked by your doctor. He or she will very probably want to run some routine tests to eliminate the possibility of an underlying condition such as anaemia or maybe an imbalanced thyroid gland function. The following advice can be an invaluable help, however, as a first

line of attack if you feel that you need to bounce your energy levels back up to the healthy side of the equation. Safe complementary measures such as the ones listed overleaf can play an immensely positive, practical role in supporting you back to a state of optimum health and vitality if you have recently gone through a period of neglecting yourself as a result of extra pressure and stress.

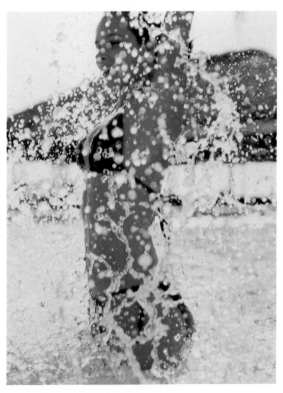

LEFT **WE ALL NEED ENOUGH ENERGY TO FACE DAILY LIFE, BUT NOT SO MUCH THAT WE CANNOT SWITCH OFF.**
RIGHT **WATER HAS POWERFULLY INVIGORATING AS WELL AS HYDRATING PROPERTIES.**

REMEDIES FOR COMMON HYPERENERGY PROBLEMS

Inability to Switch Off

The inability to switch off can be one of the most infuriating and common side effects of having a high-pressure lifestyle. If you extend your working boundaries further and further, and leave little time to yourself within which to unwind and relax, you are almost certainly going to have problems switching off effectively when you need to.

There are specific behavioural habits we may be tempted to adopt that only make things worse in the long run, such as relying on alcohol or sedative painkillers. These won't give you a pleasurable sense of being relaxed and clear-headed, but are far more likely to leave you feeling drowsy and slightly spaced out. Try the following measures instead of reaching for the easy option. They should help you to switch off when you need to, without compromising your basic sense of energy and vitality.

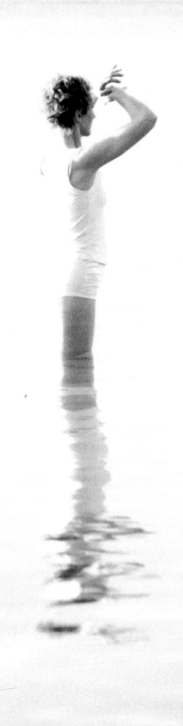

Autogenic Training

- **Consider a course in autogenic training; this is a simple but effective system of switching off that teaches you how to achieve a state of deep relaxation.**

- **When you initially set about learning the basics of this technique, it's best to be taught by a trained practitioner, rather than trying to teach yourself.**

- **Once you've mastered the basics, autogenic training can be switched on to trigger a profoundly relaxed state within a relatively short space of time. Most important of all, this technique is very simple and can be practised anywhere without any paraphernalia or fuss.**

Yoga

- **Learning yoga will teach you how to use your breathing to stimulate a sense of increased energy or a profoundly relaxed state, depending on your individual needs at any given time, and the postures will enable you to achieve inner and outer stillness. You can benefit hugely from regular practice if you want to switch off effectively.**

- If you are a beginner, make sure that you attend classes run by a fully qualified practitioner.

Meditation

- If you find that you can't just switch off the chattering in your mind, learning a simple meditation technique can help you to turn on the relaxation response when required.

- For a simple meditation exercise, sit in a straight-backed chair in a quiet, comfortable room. Empty your mind consciously of distracting thoughts by focusing on an image. This could be an actual object placed in front of you (e.g. a lighted candle or a flower), or it could be an image you generate in your mind. If distracting thoughts intrude – and they are bound to at first – don't become disheartened and give up. Instead, mentally push the unwanted thoughts gently to one side, and refocus your attention on your chosen image.

Panic Attacks

There is nothing quite as energy draining as being in a constant state of anxiety. If you also experience occasional panic attacks when the pressure is on, you may eventually reach a state of total emotional, mental and physical exhaustion.

But there is good news. The following three alternative and complementary therapies can all be employed to induce a state of relaxation during times of stress. Apart from making you less prone to panic attacks, they also put you in the important position of knowing that you will be able to take effective action whenever tension levels build.

Aromatherapy

- Studies have shown that aromatherapy has important mood-balancing and stress-reducing effects when used as part of a general complementary approach to healing mind and body. When harnessed in combination with massage, essential oils appear to play a significant role in relieving accumulated mental, emotional and physical tensions and anxiety.

LEFT **PRACTISING BEING IN THE MOMENT CAN PROVE A SURPRISINGLY EFFECTIVE STRESSBUSTER.**

- To relieve a panic attack, a few drops of any of the following essential oils can either be inhaled from a tissue or defused in a custom-made vaporizer: **bergamot, ylang ylang, lavender, clary sage, frankincense.**

Herbal Help

- Persistently low energy levels that are the result of nervous exhaustion may respond well to taking a course of **avena sativa** tincture. Made from wild oats in a liquid suspension of alcohol, eight drops of tincture in a small glass of water should be taken each day for a month. The course can be repeated if anxiety levels begin to escalate again.

- To help you to 'chill out' when the heat is on tablets that contain a combination of **hops** and **valerian** can be an invaluable aid. **Valerian,** especially, appears to be an all-round anxiety reliever, treating rising levels of agitation and sleeplessness without the attendant drowsiness and muzzy-headedness that are common side effects of conventional tranquillizers.

Homeopathy

- Anxiety and blind panic that descend on you rapidly and abruptly may be eased swiftly and effectively with a dose or two of **aconite**. This can also be an invaluable remedy in reducing anxiety that is a response to severe shock or trauma (e.g. being involved in an accident or receiving bad news).

- 'Free-floating' anxiety that attaches itself to anything that is mildly worrying can be considerably eased by a few doses of **phosphorus**. People who respond well to this remedy tend to be very outgoing, sociable and sensitive to the moods and needs of others. The downside of this very reactive, creative temperament is that they can quickly become drained of emotional and physical energy, so that they rapidly feel exhausted and apathetic.

- Anxiety that takes the form of a mental and emotional 'short fuse' with lots of anxious irritability, tension headaches and severe insomnia may be noticeably relieved by a dose or two of **nux vomica**. Confirmatory symptoms include reliance on coffee, alcohol and cigarettes in order to keep up with a punishing pace of work and play.

Insomnia

We all need regular, refreshing sleep as a cornerstone of vibrant health and vitality. Once you are in more than a short-term phase of disturbed sleep, you pay a high price in the form of mental and physical fatigue, mood swings, susceptibility to minor infections and cosmetic nuisances such as black, puffy circles under your eyes. The following gentle nonaddictive complementary measures should help you to break the negative sleep cycle in double-quick time.

Aromatherapy
- Try vaporizing a few drops of any of the following sleep-inducing oils in a custom-made vaporizer in your bedroom before retiring. Choose from these three: **lavender, camomile, ylang ylang.**

- Alternatively, a drop or two of your chosen oil can be put on a tissue and kept near your pillow.

Herbal Help
- Herbal preparations that include **valerian** can help you to relax at night without any of the drawbacks associated with conventional sleeping tablets. Adverse effects of the latter can include a slightly 'hungover' feeling on waking that lasts through the first half of the day and a risk of developing a dependency on the medication. This can lead to the need for increasingly higher doses to be taken in order to reproduce the initial effect.

Homeopathy
- Short-term insomnia that follows delayed shock of bad news or an accident can be relieved by a few doses of **aconite.** Fast acting, this remedy is needed if you toss and turn in bed as the result of a constant state of physical, mental and emotional restlessness.

- **Aconite** can also help to banish nightmares that cause you to wake suddenly in a blind panic.

- Recent sleep problems that have descended as a result of short-term anxiety about meeting high or extra-challenging standards at work may be better resolved with a few doses of **arsenicum album.** Confirmatory symptoms indicating a need for this remedy include a specific tendency to wake some time after midnight (characteristically at around 2 am), especially if wakefulness is accompanied by a strong sense of anxiety, restlessness and chilliness.

- If you are addicted to living life in the fast lane but 'crash and burn' and frequently have associated problems in getting a sound or refreshing night's sleep, you are almost certainly going to have success with a few doses of **nux vomica.** This remedy is especially useful if you habitually rely on stimulants (caffeinated drinks such as coffee, tea and colas) to keep up with the pace, and alcohol and cigarettes to wind down. Overuse of these props will make switching off in bed pretty impossible to achieve, and incur a tendency to feel hungover, heavy-headed and grouchy when you wake up in the morning.

Tension Headaches

Recurrent tension headaches do very little for your mood, ability to concentrate and overall sense of vitality. Tell-tale symptoms include pain located at the back of the head or that radiates from the base of the skull to above the eyes. Your neck, shoulders and jaw are also likely to feel clenched and taut, too, with your shoulders often being raised a few inches upwards towards your ears. This tense position can sadly make the pain and discomfort worse, as it has the negative effect of restricting blood flow to the muscles of the head and scalp.

If you suffer from tension headaches, you may be inadvertently aggravating the condition by taking painkillers such as combination codeine and paracetamol formulas. Although medication of this kind can appear to ease the pain of tension headaches effectively in the short term, it can make the situation worse in the long run by triggering 'rebound' headaches.

The following gentle but effective alternative and complementary measures are well worth trying when you experience the first twinge of pain associated with a tension headache, and they may even help to ward off a full-scale attack.

Aromatherapy

- Dilute four drops of **peppermint** essential oil in a tablespoon of carrier oil, and apply the soothing blend on a cotton bud (Q-Tip) to the area along the edge of the hairline. Alternatively, drop a few drops of **peppermint** essential oil on a tissue and inhale (avoiding the neat oil making contact with the tip of your nose).

- For women whose tension headaches are markedly worse premenstrually, a couple of drops of **clary sage** diluted in a carrier oil and applied to the hairline in the way described above may be helpful.

Instant Relaxation

- The next time the first twinge of a tension headache threatens, bring your attention to how your jaw feels. It is probably clenched firmly shut without your having been conscious of this. You may also find that you wake up with a similar tight sensation in the jaw and your partner may have noticed that you grind your teeth in your sleep. If this is the case, the following simple relaxation technique is well worth trying whenever the pressure is building.

BELOW **REFRESHING SLEEP IS NATURE'S BALM AND A PLEASURABLE WAY OF RECHARGING YOUR BATTERIES.**

- Consciously relax the muscles of your face and jaw, deliberately focusing your attention on letting go of any tension held in the muscles of your shoulders and arms. You should find as you do this that your lips part a little quite naturally and your shoulders drop an inch or two down from your ears. Concentrate on keeping all the muscles in your arms relaxed. As you grow used to doing this effectively, your fingers should naturally curl slightly inwards as they are held less rigidly.

Herbal Help

- A calming infusion of tension-busting **lime flower**, **camomile** or **lemon verbena** can help diffuse a tension headache that is the body's response to a period of high stress and pressure.

Homeopathy

- Tension headaches that come on after a combination of late nights, too much stress and an excess of caffeine can be soothed by a dose or two of **coffea**. Confirmatory symptoms include oversensitivity to the slightest noise, a constant flow of ideas that refuse to be switched off and a sharp, one-sided headache that feels as though a nail is being driven into the site of the pain. Eating makes the headache worse, while lying peacefully in a quiet, dark room is soothing.

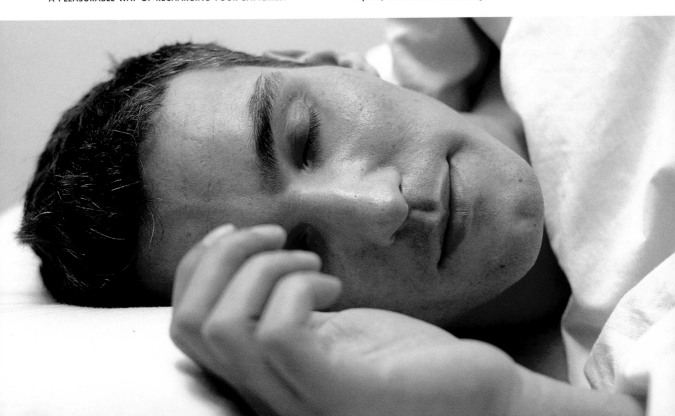

- Left-sided tension headaches that come on after sleep may respond to **lachesis**. In this situation, the pain may be instantly relieved by the onset of a natural discharge (e.g. a running nose or the beginning of a period), while it worsens with feeling overheated and hemmed in.

- Right-sided tension headaches with marked sensitivity of the muscles of the scalp and pain that is made much more intense by even the slightest movement may be quickly soothed by a few doses of **bryonia**.

Water Therapy

- Tension headaches can be aggravated by a low-level state of dehydration that can lead to constipation, which will further increase the risk of headaches developing. This is why maintaining adequate water intake is vital.

Massage

- If tension headaches are a well-established problem and the tension in your head, face, neck and shoulders feels like armour-plating, investing in a course of professional treatment to get you well on the way to recovery is a wise move, not just a luxury. Consider having a regular neck and back treatment, or an Indian head massage.

Mood Swings

Subtle mood swings are a basic part and parcel of life as we react to whatever punches life may throw at us from time to time. Normally, they are nothing to worry about nor are they indicative of a deeper problem. On the other hand, more severe or erratic mental and emotional reactions do deserve attention if they appear to be forming a regular or frequent pattern. Apart from the unpleasant feeling of not being in control of your life, recurrent mood swings can make you feel downright exhausted as you attempt to cope with being flung about on an emotional roller coaster.

Common triggers of mood swings can include hormonal fluctuations or imbalances (due to puberty, premenstrual syndrome, menopause, pregnancy, thyroid imbalance or male menopause), or high stress levels that are not being managed effectively. Severe mood swings can also be symptomatic of underlying struggles with chronic anxiety and even depression. If this is the case, professional medical help should be sought as early as possible in order to obtain the necessary support you will need to make a good recovery.

On the other hand, if your mood swings seem to be just part of a general condition of feeling 'burnt out' as the result of keeping your foot on the accelerator pedal of your life for a bit too long, the following alternative and complementary measures should help you to apply the brakes.

BELOW **A HEAD, NECK AND SHOULDER MASSAGE CAN DO WONDERS FOR RELEASING BUILT-UP MUSCULAR TENSION.**

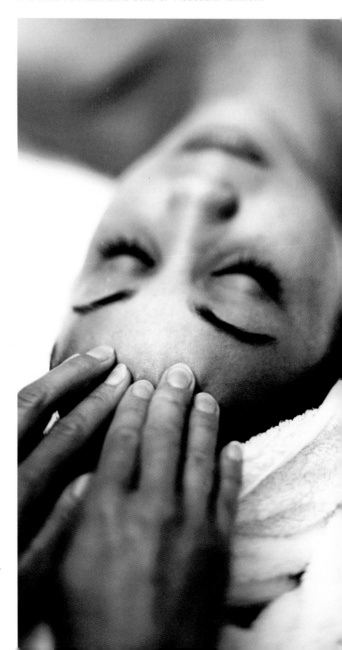

Nutritional Balance

- The quality and frequency of what you eat and drink can have a considerable effect on mood swings. This is mainly owing to the way that fluctuating levels of blood sugar can trigger any of the following: poor concentration, irritability, jitteriness, slight dizziness, muzzy-headedness and fatigue. If you have an underlying tendency to fairly volatile changes of mood, it is important to make a point of keeping your blood sugar levels as stable as possible (see also below).

- Have something small to eat every two to three hours. Choose items that are digested slowly such as wholemeal (wholewheat) crackers, wholemeal (wholewheat) bread or a small piece of fruit.

- Avoid items that cause erratic fluctuations in blood sugar. Major offenders are coffee, tea, chocolate, biscuits (cookies), anything made from white flour and white sugar, and carbonated sweetened drinks.

- Don't make the mistake of going for hours without anything to eat or drink, however busy you may be. It's sure to do nothing in the long run for your sense of equilibrium or your concentration.

- If problems with mood swings are severe or well established, and you are fairly sure that dietary factors are implicated in some way, it's worth consulting a trained nutritionist for expert advice.

Nutritional Supplements

- **Vitamin B complex** is a water-soluble vitamin that can do a great deal to support your nervous system when a crisis hits. It can be a good option to take a course if you feel that your moods are suffering under stress.

- If you're prone to attacks of the 'blues' from time to time, consider a course of **sam-e**. A compound that occurs naturally in our bodies through a process called methylation, sam-e appears to have a beneficial effect on low mood while reducing symptoms of painful joints and muscles. No adverse side effects have been reported in clinical trials, and the recommended starting dose is 200 mg twice daily.

Aromatherapy

- A few drops of any of the following essential oils can be vaporized as an effective and pleasurable way of balancing fraught moods and promoting a general sense of wellbeing: **ylang ylang**, **rose**, **neroli**, **mandarin**.

- Aromatherapy massages may also lift your spirits, and you will usually be able to select from several blends of oils.

Aerobic Exercise

- Get those feel-good chemicals moving in your system by making a point of taking regular exercise that conditions the heart and lungs. Suitable choices include cycling, running, power walking, swimming and dancing. Regularity is a must if it is to work: aim for three or four 45-minute sessions each week.

Herbal Help

- **Rhodiola** is classed as an adaptogen that appears to stabilize mood, boost overall immunity and improve concentration. The suggested dose is 200–300 mg daily taken with food.

Homeopathy

- Rapidly changing moods that have set in after an emotionally distressing experience (e.g. break-up of a relationship, bereavement or loss of a job) may be eased greatly by a short course of **ignatia**. This is a rapidly acting remedy that should promote a perceptible stabilizing of mood within a few days. Once this has happened, no more of the remedy is needed, unless or until symptoms show signs of recurring.

- Mood swings that have an obvious hormonal trigger (e.g. following pregnancy, premenstrually or during menopause) may be considerably reduced by a few doses of **pulsatilla**. Classic symptoms that suggest this remedy is needed include frequent weepiness, a craving for comfort, sympathy and attention, and a general sense of being hugely better for a good cry.

- **Sepia** is immensely helpful when there is a general sense of mental, emotional and physical flatness, combined with a sense of being wound-up and unable to cope with any more demands. This negative spiral often sets in as a

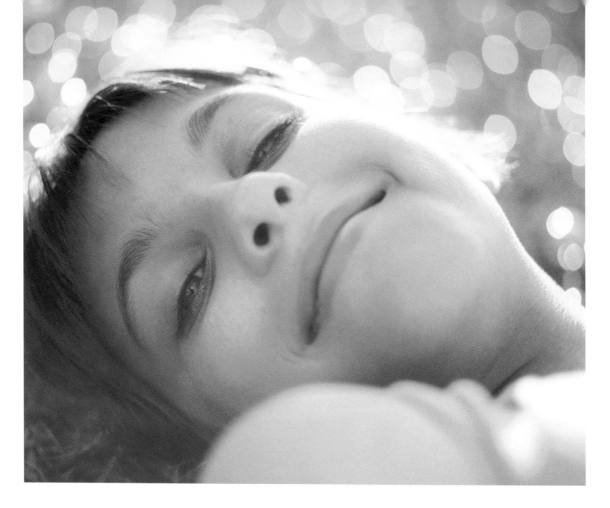

reaction to accumulated stress and pressure. This remedy can restore a flagging or nonexistent libido and also re-establish general emotional and physical vitality.

Light Therapy

- If you wrestle each winter with feelings of moodiness, negativity and sluggishness, plus a general desire to hibernate until spring comes around again, you may do well to consider investing in some full-spectrum lighting. This mimics the effect of natural sunlight and appears to benefit those who suffer with seasonal affective disorder (SAD).

ME (Myalgic Encephalomyelitis)

ME is a debilitating condition that is classed as a chronic problem. In other words, it doesn't occur as a one-off episode of illness, but has a tendency to develop into a long-term affliction with repeated flare-ups of symptoms being a common feature.

Controversy has long raged within the medical establishment over whether ME really exists, but a

ABOVE SENSIBLE EXPOSURE TO SUNLIGHT CAN DO A GREAT DEAL TO LIFT FLAGGING SPIRITS. IN DARK WINTER MONTHS, YOU CAN TRY LIGHT THERAPY TO MIMIC THE SUN.

recent British government report recognized it to be a serious illness and called for faster diagnosis and improved treatment. Today it is generally accepted as a genuine illness.

Symptoms of ME are extremely distressing and may include any combination of the following:

- Incapacitating exhaustion that often prevents the sufferer getting out of bed
- Muscle aches and pains
- Poor memory and concentration
- Anxiety
- Depression
- Sleep problems
- Sweating
- Headaches
- Thrush (*Candida albicans*)
- Swollen glands

- Digestive problems including stomach cramps and diarrhoea

The severity of these symptoms varies from one person to another; some may experience a broad range of symptoms, but others just a few. Causes and triggers of the condition are numerous, but each of the following is a possibility:

- A severe viral illness with insufficient time allowed to convalesce
- Damaged immunity from overuse of antibiotics
- An adverse reaction to vaccination
- Too stressful a lifestyle with insufficient or unhealthy coping mechanisms

This illness most commonly hits those between the ages of 15 and 40, with women being more frequently affected than men. It has also been suggested that those of us who are high achievers, who tend to cut ourselves too little slack within which to rest and recuperate after illness, may also be more vulnerable to this condition.

As tricky as ME can sometimes be to diagnose and treat (there is not yet any specific test that can be performed to confirm a diagnosis of ME), the good news is that alternative and complementary measures can be an immensely valuable source of support and can aid recovery. As this is a chronic condition and complicated case management can be called for, it's important to seek professional alternative medical treatment from a properly qualified practitioner to give yourself the maximum chance of a positive outcome. Any of the following therapies can help:

- Aromatherapy
- Homeopathy
- Osteopathy
- Nutritional therapy
- Remedial yoga therapy
- Western medical herbalism
- Naturopathy
- Counselling for stress management
- Traditional Chinese medicine

REMEDIES FOR COMMON HYPO-ENERGY PROBLEMS

Persistent Fatigue

Reaching a state of constant tiredness is usually the end result of a number of common triggers that can be an intrinsic part of 21st-century living. They may include any combination of the following:

- Poor stress management at times of pressure
- Reliance on junk foods and stimulants
- Lack of good-quality sleep
- The after-effects of a severe viral illness
- Irregular eating
- A sedentary lifestyle

Unfortunately, you're likely to find that one factor will impact on another, leading to a negative spiral of tiredness that keeps going downwards, becoming a little more severe all the time. So, for instance, if you take very little exercise, you may find that you don't sleep well or soundly. As a result, you are very likely to rely on quick fixes when you start the day (lots of sugar and caffeine) to raise your low energy levels. This only leads to a further slump of energy further later on, and the stimulants in your body contribute to another disturbed night.

The secrets of breaking this vicious, energy-depleting circle are contained in each chapter of this book – you can choose the area in which you want to get started. But if you want a quick booster to get you through a temporary patch of tiredness, the ideas below should get you off to a good start. Don't be misled into thinking that you can cheat by resorting to a quick fix in this way on an ongoing basis: you still need to put in place the basic energy building blocks if you don't want to come to grief a little further on down the line.

Aromatherapy
- **A few drops of any of the following essential oils may be burnt in a custom-made vaporizer or inhaled from a tissue when energy levels are in need of a boost: grapefruit, lemon, orange, peppermint, rosemary.**

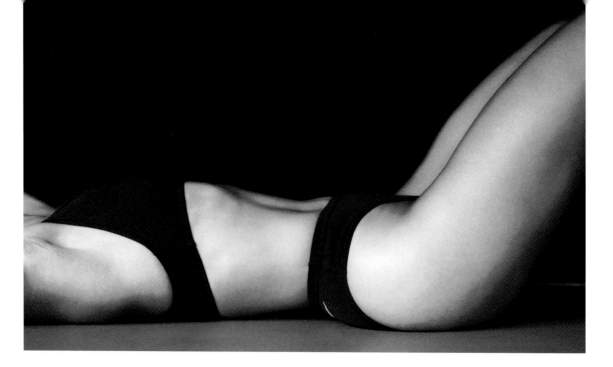

Exercise

- If your problems stem from working at a desk all day, driving home and spending the evening in front of the television or on the Internet, it's time to take a gentle but firm look at how you can become more active. If you like a reflective approach, excellent energy-balancing systems of movement include **hatha yoga, t'ai chi** and **chi gong**. If you know you would prefer fast-paced movement, opt instead for **cycling** (either outdoors or on a static exercise bike), **running, ashtanga yoga, Tae Bo** or **racket sports**.

Homeopathy

- If your energy levels are sluggish and low after too many nights on the town when you've eaten too much junk food, had too many late nights and consumed far too much alcohol, with a hefty dose of caffeine thrown in for good measure, **nux vomica** is just what you need while you clean up your act. This remedy is a major detoxifier, and a few doses can have you feeling human again within a day or two, and ready to get your life back in order by kicking the late nights, alcohol and junk food. If you're a party person, always have some nux vomica on hand.

- If your energy levels are still sluggish after putting energy-boosting, self-help measures into action, consider consulting a qualified homeopathic practitioner who will be able to look at the overall picture with a trained, objective eye.

ABOVE APPROPRIATE EXERCISE CAN IMPROVE STRENGTH, STAMINA AND FLEXIBILITY ENORMOUSLY, AS WELL AS ENCOURAGING A LEANER BODY.

Other East-West Therapies

- You may find it helpful to explore other systems of alternative medicine, including **Western medical herbalism, ayurvedic medicine** and **traditional Chinese medicine**. If you suspect that your energy levels are being drained by constantly holding muscles in a tight, tense posture, the **Alexander Technique** or a course of **aromatherapy massage** may be helpful.

Nutritional Therapy

- **Ginseng** has a well-known reputation as a general vitality-boosting adaptogen. Clinical trials suggest that it provides support for our bodies when they are exposed to emotional and physical stress and pressure. As a result, mental and physical energy levels appear to improve, as well as overall stamina, concentration and resilience. Always avoid the bargain option when buying **ginseng**, as the quality of the product is the key to achieving positive results. Cheaper products may actually contain very little of the active ingredient. The optimum suggested dose is 200 mg twice daily, taken in split doses of 100 mg each. As with many supplements, it's best to avoid taking ginseng on a routine basis. Instead, take it in occasional two-weekly courses, whenever become aware that your energy levels are flagging.

- Thought to boost the energy and immune system, **co-enzyme Q10** has been christened the 'spark of life'. It is an important antioxidant nutrient, and possible dietary sources include oily fish (e.g. sardines and mackerel), offal and peanuts. Sadly, it is thought that it is difficult to receive enough of this antioxidant through our daily intake of food to be therapeutically effective. So if energy levels plummet as a result of any of the vitality-draining lifestyle factors listed previously, consider taking a course of co-enzyme Q10. This can give your body a general boost while you eliminate those energy-draining aspects from your daily life.

Weight Gain

Reaching an optimum weight these days is an extremely fraught and complex matter. The situation isn't made any easier by images of stick-thin supermodels confronting us constantly in the glossy magazines, the latest diet fad convincing us that we will be slimmer, more desirable, more successful and happier if we lose weight according to its rules, and a society that generally sets ever more store by appearances and is seemingly intolerant of anything outside the so-called norm.

All these factors can conspire towards making you more concerned about gaining a few extra pounds than you should be. On the other hand, if you are genuinely worried about carrying so much extra weight that it restricts your life and makes it uncomfortable and difficult to climb a flight of stairs without becoming breathless, then it is time to take positive action to improve your health and fitness – for you, though, not for someone else's notion of how you should be.

As far as assessing whether you are genuinely overweight or not, you are far better off discarding tables that tell you what your ideal weight is and much better off working out how you feel at the weight that you are. Any of the following questions will be of more value than relying on weight assessment tables alone.

- Is your breathing laboured or heavy after you have run a short distance?

- Do you feel noticeably out of breath when climbing a couple of flights of stairs at a fairly brisk pace?
- Does your clothing feel uncomfortably tight and restrictive after a fairly short time?
- Are there any visible signs of excess flesh on your upper arms, belly, hips and/or thighs?
- Do you feel sluggish and disinclined to join an exercise class because it's such an effort to get moving?

If you've answered yes to most of these questions, there is a strong chance that losing some weight will be beneficial to your overall health and sense of

BELOW **WEIGHING SCALES CAN ONLY TELL YOU SO MUCH ABOUT WHETHER YOU ARE OVERWEIGHT OR NOT. HOW HEALTHY AND AT EASE WE FEEL IN OUR BODIES IS JUST AS IMPORTANT AS HOW HEAVY WE ARE.**

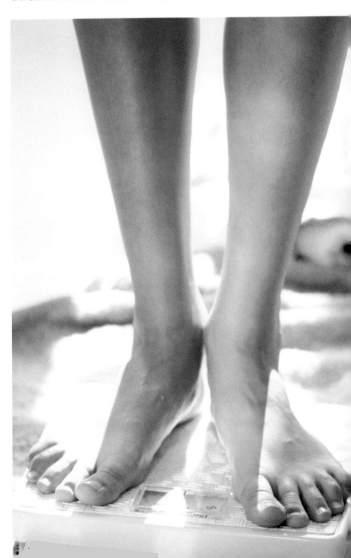

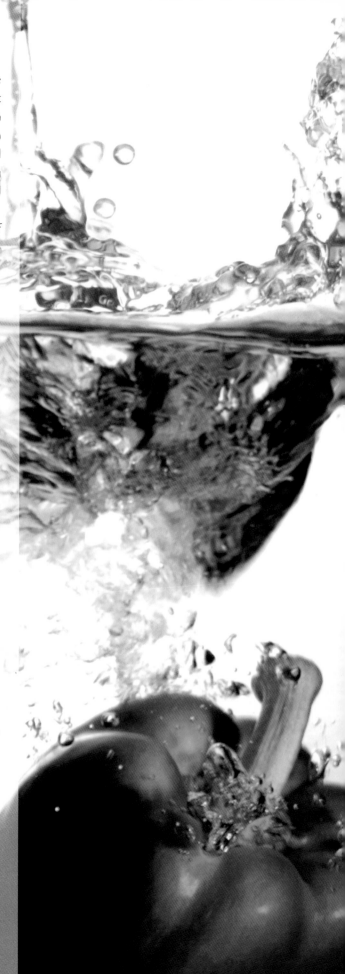

wellbeing. On the other hand, if you weigh more than is recommended by an ideal-weight table but feel perfectly fit and healthy, there may be no reason to take radical weight-reducing steps. This is even more the case if your subjective impression is backed up by medical tests that assess your heart rate, lung capacity, blood pressure, cholesterol levels and blood sugar readings.

Being genuinely overweight can lead to some of the following problems, so it is clearly something to guard against for health reasons:

- Increased risk of type II diabetes
- Heart disease
- High blood pressure
- Joint problems such as osteoarthritis
- Varicose veins
- Lack of self-esteem and confidence
- Constant fatigue

For established weight problems, you should ideally consult a trained practitioner in any of the following alternative and complementary disciplines who will be in the best position to advise you on how healthily to reach an optimum weight and stay there:

- Ayurvedic medicine
- Homeopathy
- Nutritional therapy
- Naturopathy

Nutritional Therapy

- If you are concerned about your weight, assess your nutrition on a daily basis to discover what foods or drinks may be the hidden culprits in your diet. Honestly evaluate the quality and quantity of what you eat and drink daily by making a list of everything that passes your lips over a 48-hour period. You may be surprised by the results.

- Make keeping a good-quality eating plan a top priority. Bear in mind that foods of low nutritional status (those containing white flour, white sugar, a high proportion of saturated fat, and additives in the form of artificial flavourings, preservatives and colourings) tend to leave you unsatisfied and ready for more within a short time.

- Exchange refined, highly processed foods for fresh foods that give you the full complement of fibre, vitamins and minerals, and small amounts of protein. Avoid full-fat cheeses, margarine, lashings of butter, fried foods and battered items. Accentuate high-fibre foods such as salads made from raw, grated or bite-sized vegetables, fresh fruit, unroasted and unsalted seeds and nuts, pulses, beans, wholemeal (wholewheat) bread and pasta, steamed brown rice, fish, and homemade soups and broths to which small portions of free-range chicken or organic meat may be added. Resist adding mayonnaise to salads; opt for a dressing made from a little cold-pressed olive oil and vinegar, or plain (natural) yoghurt.

- At all costs, avoid faddy, yo-yo dieting. Drastic weight loss at any time makes you more likely to pile the weight back on once you go back to your normal eating patterns. Sadly, there's every chance that you'll gain even more weight the second time around, as your body reacts to having been in starvation mode by lowering your metabolic rate. Also avoid like the plague diets that go against what we now know to be sound nutritional guidelines (this includes soup diets, fluid-restrictive diets and diets high in saturated animal fats). These may stimulate weight loss, but at great cost to your overall health. In other words: if it's drastic, don't do it.

Sluggish Digestion

A digestive system that frequently functions in a less than efficient way can burden you with a host of problems that have an adverse effect on your basic energy levels. After all, it's very hard to feel as though you're bouncing with vitality if you're suffering from severe indigestion or a bout of constipation. As well as getting your dietary act back into good shape, alternative and complementary medicines can do a great deal to help shift your digestive system up to a higher gear. Some of the most simple and practical measures which should yield positive results within a day or so are listed here. However, always seek

LEFT ALWAYS SCRUB OR THOROUGHLY WASH FRUIT AND VEGETABLES BEFORE CHOPPING OR COOKING, WHETHER THEY ARE FROM ORGANIC OR NONORGANIC SOURCES.

medical advice if your digestive problems prove resistant to self-help measures or if you notice any unexplained change in stomach or bowel habits.

Herbal Help

- Discomfort and flatulence that follow overindulgence can be soothed by an infusion of **peppermint** or **fennel tea**. Be prepared to experience a lot of wind once it's drunk.

- General queasiness can be swiftly relieved by sucking a piece of crystallized **ginger**. Alternatively, a similar but less sweet effect can be obtained by slowly sipping a warming cup of **ginger** tea.

- Acidity that sets in after a heavy meal can be banished by a hot drink made by dissolving two generous teaspoons of **slippery elm** powder in a cup of hot milk. Slippery elm bark taken in powdered form has a reputation for reducing irritation of the stomach lining.

- **Aloe vera** has attracted a great deal of positive attention owing to its reputation for soothing the digestive tract and encouraging regular bowel movements. Thankfully it appears to be able to do this without the problems of dependency and malabsorption associated with conventional antacids and laxatives.

Homeopathy

- Simple cases of indigestion with lots of burping and flatulence, with a troublesome heavy, overfull sensation in the stomach and bloating around the belly, may be cleared up quickly with a dose or two of **carbo veg**.

- Stubborn constipation that develops as a result of low-level dehydration, with a dull, 'toxic' headache and short-fused mood may be considerably eased by two or three doses of **bryonia**.

Water Therapy

- Many of us are now aware of the need for high-fibre foods in our diets, but we are often unaware that a high percentage of constipation difficulties are due to low-level dehydration. To remedy this, make a point of drinking five large glasses of filtered or still mineral water, spaced evenly throughout the day.

Recommended Reading

Agombar, Fiona, *Endless Energy: Over Fifty Ways to Fight Fatigue*, Piatkus, 2002

Alexander, Jane, *The Energy Secret: Practical Techniques for Understanding and Directing Vital Energy*, Thorsons, 2000

Brewer, Dr Sarah, *The Total De-Tox Plan: A Comprehensive Program to Cleanse Your Mind and Body*, Carlton Books, 2002

Downing-Orr, Dr Kristina, *What to Do If You're Burned Out and Blue: The Essential Guide to Help You Through Depression*, Thorsons, 2000

Fonda, Jane, *Women Coming of Age*, Viking, 1985

Kenton, Leslie, *Boost Energy*, Vermillion, 1996

Kenton, Susannah and Leslie, *Endless Energy: For Women on the Move*, Vermillion, 1993

Kenton, Susannah and Leslie, *The New Raw Energy*, Vermillion, 1994

Lalvani, Vimla, *Yoga: The Total Yoga Workout for Mind, Body and Spirit*, Hamlyn, 1999

Lavery, Sheila, *The Healing Power of Sleep: How to Achieve Restorative Sleep Naturally*, Gaia, 1997

MacEoin, Beth, *Natural Medicine: A Practical Guide to Family Health*, Bloomsbury, 1999

MacEoin, Beth, *The Total De-Stress Plan: A Complete Guide to Working with Positive and Negative Stress*, Carlton Books, 2002

Morrison, Judith, *The Book of Ayurveda: A Guide to Personal Wellbeing*, Gaia, 1994

Petersen-Schepelern, Elsa, *Smoothies and Other Blended Drinks*, Ryland, Peters and Small, 1996

Simon, David, MD, *Vital Energy: The Seven Keys to Invigorate Body, Mind and Soul*, John Wiley and Sons, 2000

Van Straten, Michael, *The Good Sleep Guide*, Kyle Cathie Limited, 1996

Vyas, Bharti, with Haggard, Claire, *Beauty Wisdom: The Secret of Looking and Feeling Fabulous*, Thorsons, 1997

Wildwood, Chrissie, *The Bloomsbury Encyclopaedia of Aromatherapy*, Bloomsbury, 1996

Address Book

UK

COMPLEMENTARY MEDICINE (GENERAL)
Council for Complementary and Alternative Medicine
Park House
206–208 Latimer Road
London W10 6RE
Tel: 020 8735 0400
www.acupuncture.org.uk

General Council and Register of Naturopaths
2 Goswell Road
Street, Somerset BA16 0JG
Tel: 01458 840072
www.naturopathy.org.uk

National Institute of Medical Herbalists
56 Longbrooke Street
Exeter EX4 8HA
Tel: 01392 426022
www.btinternet.com/-nimh

The Society of Homeopaths
2 Artizan Road
Northampton NN1 4HU
Tel: 01604 621400
www.homeopathy-soh.org

BODYWORK
Aromatherapy Organisations Council
PO Box 19834
London SE25 6WF
Tel: 020 8251 7912
www.aromatherapy-uk.org

British Acupuncture Council
Park House
206–208 Latimer Road
London W10 6RE
Tel: 020 8735 0400
www.acupuncture.org.uk

British Massage Therapy Council
17 Rymers Lane
Oxford OX4 3JU
Tel: 01865 774123
www.bmtc.co.uk

Society of Teachers of the Alexander Technique
129 Camden Mews
London NW1 9AH
Tel: 020 7284 3338
www.stat.org.uk

EXERCISE
Body Control Pilates Association
14 Neals Yard
London WC2H 9DP
Tel: 020 7379 3734
www.bodycontrol.co.uk

British Wheel of Yoga
1 Hamilton Place
Boston Road, Sleaford
Lincolnshire NG34 7ES
Tel: 01529 306851
www.bwy.org.uk

The Pilates Foundation
80 Camden Road
London E17 7NF
Tel: 07071 781859
www.pilatesfoundation.com

T'ai chi Union of Great Britain
94 Felsham Road
London SW15 1DQ
Tel: 020 8780 1063
Email: comptonph@aol.com

Tse Qi Gong Centre
Tel: 01619 294485
www.bodytao.co.uk

NUTRITION
The Institute for
Optimum Nutrition
13 Blades Court
Deodar Road
London SW15 2NU
Tel: 020 8877 9993

The Nutri Centre
The Hale Clinic
7 Park Crescent
London W1N 3HE
Tel: 020 7436 5122
www.nutricentre.com

USA

Alexander Technique Center
Email: info@alexandercenter.com
www.alexandercenter.com

American Association
of Acupuncture and
Oriental Medicine
4101 Lake Boone
Trail Suite 201
Raleigh, NC 27607
Tel: 919 787 5181
www.holisticmedicine.com

American Chiropractic
Association
1701 Clarendon Blvd
Arlington, VA 22209

Tel: 703 276 8800
www.acatoday.com

American Herbalist Guild
1931 Gaddis Road
Canton, GA 30115
Tel: 770 751 6021
www.americanherbalistguild.com

Body/Mind Restoration Retreats
56 Lieb Road
Spencer, NY 14883
Tel: 607 272 0694
ww.bodymindretreats.com

International Association
of Yoga Therapists
2400A County Center Drive
Santa Rosa, CA 95403
Tel: 707 566 9000
www.iayt.org

The National Association
for Holistic Aromatherapy
4509 Interlake Avenue
North Seattle, WA 98103–6773
Tel: 206 547 2164
www.naha.org

National Certification Board
for Therapeutic Massage and
Bodywork
8201 Greensboro Drive
Suite 300
McLean, VA 22102
Tel: 800 296 0664
www.ncbtmb.com

National Institute of
Ayurvedic Medicine
584 Milltown Road
Brewster, New York 10509
Tel: 845 274 8700
Fax: 845 278 8251

Nutritional Center for Homeopathy
801 North Fairfax Street
Suite 306
Alexandria, VA 22314
Tel: 703 548 7790
www.homeopathy.org

CANADA

Acupuncture Canada
107 Leitch Drive
Grimsby
Ontario L3M 2T9
Tel: 905 563 8930
www.acupuncture.ca

The Canadian Herb Society
5251 Oak Street
Vancouver
British Columbia V6M 4H1
www.herbsociety.ca

Tzu Chi Institute for
Complementary Medicine
767 West 12th Avenue
Vancouver
British Columbia V5Z 1M9
Tel: 604 875 4769
www.tzu-chi.ba.ca

AUSTRALIA

Association of Traditional
Health Practitioners Inc.
PO Box 346
Elizabeth
South Australia 5112
Tel: 08 8284 2324
Www.traditionalmedicine.net.au

Australian Homeopathic
Association
PO Box 396
Drummoyne
New South Wales 2047
Tel: 02 9719 2793

National Herbalist
Association of Australia
33 Reserve Street
Annandale
New South West 2038
Tel: 02 9560 7077
www.nhaa.org.au

INDEX

Figures in italics refer to captions.

ACKNOWLEDGEMENTS

Picture credits

Every effort has been made to acknowledge correctly and contact the source and/or copyright holder of each picture, and Carlton Books Limited apologises for any unintentional errors or omissions which will be corrected in future editions of this book.

Alamy Images 55, 59, 62, 63, 84, 100, 118, 120, 122
Camera Press 102, 103
Carlton Books 1, 19, 24, 25, 26, 32, 34l, 34r, 42, 44, 45, 54, 56, 57, 65, 71, 73, 78, 90, 91, 92, 115
Corbis 13, 74
David Loftus 58, 66, 69
Flowerphotos 101
Getty Images 4, 6, 9, 10, 11, 12, 14, 16, 17, 18, 21, 22, 27, 28, 29, 31, 33, 35, 36, 39, 41, 47, 49, 50, 51, 52, 67, 68, 70, 86, 88, 90, 93, 109, 110, 112, 116, 121
Photonica 38, 61, 76, 80, 83, 96
Science Photo Library 20, 37
Scope Beauty 79, 87, 95, 98, 104, 106, 111
Vang/Rudolph Productions 48, 65

Author Acknowledgements

My warmest thanks are due to all of the following who each played an important role in transforming this book from a vague idea to a concrete reality.

Without my agent Teresa Chris this book would never have seen the light of day, since the original concept was hers. Judith More helped me to develop the basic concept further with her incisive and sensitive comments and attention, while Zia Mattocks and Siobhan O'Connor have done a splendid job in fine-tuning the manuscript with good grace and charm.

At home, as always, I have had the support of my extraordinary husband Denis. Always ready to proofread the manuscript an extra time, providing extra ideas for picture captions, not grumbling when yet another weekend has been taken up with putting final touches to the text, and lightening frustrating moments with his off-the-wall sense of humour: for all of this I give him not just my thanks, but all my love.